M000106814

7 STEPS TO STRONG

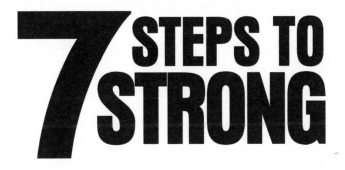

7 STEPS TO STRONG

LISA LANCEFORD

WITH ROMANE LANCEFORD

CENTURY

1 3 5 7 9 10 8 6 4 2

Century
20 Vauxhall Bridge Road
London SW1V 2SA

Century is part of the Penguin Random House group of companies whose
addresses can be found at global.penguinrandomhouse.com.

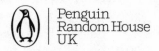

Penguin
Random House
UK

Copyright © Liro Fitness LLC 2021

Lisa Lanceford and Romane Lanceford have asserted their right to be identified
as the authors of this Work in accordance with the Copyright, Designs and
Patents Act 1988.

First published by Century in 2021

www.penguin.co.uk

A CIP catalogue record for this book is available from the British Library.

ISBN 9781529135800

Printed and bound in Great Britain by Clays Ltd, Elcograf S.p.A.

The authorised representative in the EEA is Penguin Random House Ireland,
Morrison Chambers, 32 Nassau Street, Dublin D02 YH68.

Penguin Random House is committed to a sustainable future for
our business, our readers and our planet. This book is made from
Forest Stewardship Council® certified paper.

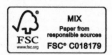

This book is dedicated to my husband,
Romane Lanceford, who gave me the gift of self-belief
and showed me anything is possible.

CONTENTS

CONTENTS

INTRODUCTION

Whenever I've thought about writing a book, or even been approached to do an interview for a website or magazine, I've always said to my husband Romane, 'Who would be interested in me?' While I've definitely suffered from self-esteem issues over the years, and I'm a pretty timid, unassuming person in general, it's not that I don't think my story is worthy – it's more that I've been lucky enough to live a relatively ordinary life without any major tragedies or trauma, and it just doesn't feel interesting enough to write about, especially when you hear the astonishing journeys that other people on social media have been on.

I grew up in a little town outside Luton in a tight-knit, traditional working-class family. My mum was a nurse, my dad was a lorry driver, and we had a huge circle of friends and family. Even now, I'm such a home girl and I hate being away from them. There was nothing particularly remarkable about my childhood – I wasn't amazing at sports and didn't really excel at school; I was always in the lowest sets and I left at sixteen with just a few crap GCSEs. I didn't have any attention-grabbing interests or talents; I just liked going out with my friends and getting drunk. Pretty ordinary, right? There was nothing to suggest that I'd go on to have a successful fitness business and become an internationally recognised influencer – it just seemed that I was destined for a steady, predictable life in Dunstable just like the rest of my family.

We live in such a connected world that I realise now how comfortable and privileged my life has been. Not that I was born with a silver spoon – from the age of sixteen I've been grafting; I worked as a hairdresser, in an electric utility company and for Network Rail – hardly the most glamorous of CVs, but I've always paid my own way. What I mean is that nothing unexpected or heartbreaking has ever happened to me, nothing which would make me feel like I should write a book. Obviously, I've had my fair share of personal challenges in relationships and trying to find my way in life, but none of it has ever felt enough to write home about.

Now, as my business has gone from strength to strength and the community around my fitness method has grown, I've started to appreciate that being a 'normal' person doesn't necessarily mean that the lessons I've learned along the way are unimportant. The truth is that there are a lot of people like me – we work hard and love our families – without our lives mirroring some dramatic plotline from a novel. That doesn't mean that what we achieve, even if it might seem small or less significant than some of the more vocal and confident people we see and hear as we scroll on our screens, is less worthy.

I wanted to write this book for women like me who aren't always the centre of attention. Perhaps like me, you spent your teens and twenties a bit lost and didn't really know which way your life was going. Perhaps you still struggle with confidence and getting your voice heard. The steps I've taken to achieve the strength I have today have been both physical and mental and have changed me massively. I always say never look at the mountain because it will just seem too far and too high to climb, but the work I've done to get to where I am has so completely improved my happiness that I feel I live a world away from my old life, and that is something I want to share with everyone.

This book relates my personal journey in seven mental and physical steps, and will hopefully inspire you to apply the same principles to your own unique situation. Of course, some of my advice is fitness- and nutrition-based because that's what I'm best known for, and I deeply believe that physical transformation can have untold positive effects on all the other areas of your life too. Fitness has definitely helped me to believe in myself and push myself to do things that I would never have done before. Weight training, in particular, has helped me to finally develop discipline, which in turn has led to confidence in myself for how far I've come. No matter what's going on in the background, no one can take away what I've achieved in the gym and weight room and that means so much to me.

One of my biggest aims is to empower you to build your own workouts and diet plans instead of prescribing a 'one size fits all' approach, which I feel is highly misleading. I want to provide you with the knowledge and the know-how to build your own plans, and after following my initial guide to sets and reps, you will able to adapt your routine to your own body goals. As part of this, I'm enlisting the help of my husband Romane, as he has an encyclopaedic understanding of physical strength. Through the seven physical steps he will explain how weightlifting actually builds your body, and which nutrients you should be eating in what quantities. He won't tell you exactly what to eat – we all have different bodies, different goals and different tastes. Some of you might be gluten- or dairy-intolerant; some of you will need more calories and some fewer, depending on your starting point. The idea of the prescriptive 'magazine diet' needs to be scrapped; we want to empower you to create a diet that works for your own unique needs and situation. Balance, moderation and knowledge beat restriction, extreme methods and confusion every time. Romane has taught me so much, and that information has had a huge impact on where I am today, so I'm thrilled to be sharing it all with you too.

What this book *isn't* about is looking a certain way, or a guide to how to lose lots of weight, because that just isn't how I think. In a way, unless you are training to compete for aesthetics, say for bodybuilding or physique, it's kind of irrelevant. Strength can look very different on different bodies, and of course the most important side of it – mental strength – is completely invisible to the naked eye. It's really about how the change makes you feel rather than numbers on a scale or what jeans size you are. While I would never discourage anyone from giving the gym a go, there are wrong and right reasons for doing it. If you're doing it to please someone else or to try to fit someone else's idea of what you should look like, it's definitely worth taking a step back and thinking about what *you* want to gain from it. For my part, I really want to emphasise how much fitness has helped me to conquer so many challenges in my life, learning some pretty hard lessons along the way. But none of them were about the way I look. And no matter how shredded my abs might look, I wouldn't be writing a book if it wasn't for the mental transformation that fitness has given me.

At the time of writing, I have 2.5 million Instagram followers and a highly engaged community of over 17,000 women in my Facebook group, all sharing their own progress stories and supporting each other in the fight to achieve their body goals. Those numbers are crazy to me, but they've made me see how many of us want to live a fuller, stronger life, and inspiring others to find the motivation, confidence and discipline to get there is what I am truly passionate about.

While I still have a lot of personal goals and ambitions, my business has fulfilled my greatest one: to help other people in some way. Seeing my mum working as a nurse and caring for people who so needed her help had a massive impact on me growing up, and now I have my own opportunity to help hundreds and thousands of women and men change their lives by getting them on a path to healthy living through training. I find my work incredibly rewarding. All I've ever wanted to do with my social accounts and fitness app is to support others like me who have struggled to change their mindset, and to be there for them on the journey to an active lifestyle. Whether it's about improving your longevity (exercise reduces your chances of hypertension, diabetes, heart disease, having a stroke ...), improving your quality of life, your relationships with others and yourself, or your motivation, exercise is one of the most powerful tools we have at our disposal – and everyone can access it.

I hope you love the workouts, my stories and life lessons, and that these seven steps to strength – both mental and physical – inspire you to start climbing your own mountains. Everyone has the potential to do amazing things, even if you're the girl or boy next door – you just have to take that first step.

Lisa x

STEP ONE TO MENTAL STRENGTH: FEMININITY IS NOT A BODY TYPE

How I found the confidence to be sexy (in my very own way)

The world of my childhood was all blue skies and fluffy white clouds. This sounds like a cliché, but it's so true. In many ways I was protected and cocooned from the outside world, and when the more negative aspects of real life invaded later on, it was a shock to my system. Of course, no one appreciates how special things are when they're young – you just think it's the norm, don't you? My immediate family are super-close and my entire family – aunties, uncles, cousins and grandparents – all lived in the same small town, Dunstable, just outside Luton. It was the quintessential suburban-town childhood, with a lot of love and support all around me; we were basically just like one big gang. That's the reason I get so homesick even to this day, and it's probably why I was such a 'young' teenager. I guess it was an old-fashioned, traditional way to be raised, and I was pretty naive, especially in comparison to the girls and women I meet in my line of work these days.

As for my immediate family, I'm the middle child with a brother either side, and my mum and dad have always had a rock-solid relationship. Both of my siblings are much more forthcoming and assertive than me, and have been ever since we were kids; I'm the softly spoken, timid middle child – people have always commented on how shy I am. When I was younger, I can remember just wanting to make my parents happy. Obviously, all teenagers push boundaries, but I was never a rebel; I think I only got two detentions in school. I always respected Mum and Dad because we were all so close as a unit. There was one time when I was about twelve and I'd been secretly smoking, and of course Mum knew – they always do, don't they? She confronted me, but she didn't shout, as my parents never shouted. Instead, she just told me how disappointed she was in me, and that absolutely killed me. I just couldn't believe I'd done that to her, and I never touched another cigarette. I so wanted to do the right thing by them that I didn't get much practice at breaking the rules or indulging in risky behaviour. I stayed within the lines and gravitated towards things that made me feel safe, a tendency that had a long-term impact on some of the decisions I made as a young woman, from the jobs I did to the boyfriends I chose.

While there was a lot of love, we definitely weren't a wealthy family, though my parents did everything they could to ensure we never felt we were missing out on anything. I know now that times were sometimes really tough for them, and when I was younger and my dad was away driving lorries, he'd be living off Mars bars because he was so skint, with all the money going to Mum to keep things together at home. I definitely wasn't raised to be materialistic, which is why possessions – from houses and cars to watches and shoes – aren't that important to me. A lot of people get into my industry to make quick money, but I've never been motivated by the financial side of things. In my younger days, if I'm honest, I wasn't really motivated by anything. I suppose you could say that, like so many other young people, I lacked direction. I didn't have any self-discipline either, which is hard to square with how regimented I can be about my routine today.

So many of the men and women I've met through my career in fitness have been incredibly driven their whole lives, and you find a lot of confident, Type-A personalities in the industry. For me, school was always about just getting by. I would never ever put my hand up or put myself forward for anything. Some of that I can put down to the type of school I went to and the teachers who squashed my confidence, but mostly it was because I was just so quiet and reserved. I was always in the bottom sets, which could be really frustrating, because I wanted to learn, and those classes were full of the clowns. It was impossible to keep focused because you were always being distracted, and you didn't get the same guidance that other classes did. That sometimes made you feel like you'd been a bit forgotten about and that your education didn't really matter. I can't say I was too bothered by the fact that I wasn't that academic though, and my family never made it seem like a big deal. There were kids in school who were really smart and would be going on to uni and all of that, but I knew that wasn't me. I always thought 'good for them' and didn't feel resentful or envious, though, because I knew that was never going to be my path. I'm so lucky that my parents never pushed anything on me, either in or out of school. They did encourage me to try extra-curricular activities, but even though I did gymnastics and ballet, nothing ever really stuck.

What was really missing from my education was any kind of advice about what I could do once I'd left. I was only sixteen when I started working and there seemed so few options available to someone like me, with rubbish GCSE grades and no money to do an unpaid internship or anything like that. My choice was literally either beauty or hairdressing, and because I was very much a girl who went with the flow and did what was expected of me, and I wasn't particularly into nails and waxing, I decided to go for hairdressing. My first job as a junior earned me £120 a week, which I'd receive in a brown paper envelope every Friday, and for that I worked ten hours nearly every single day 8am–6pm with barely a break to wolf down a sandwich. The salon was just down the road from my parents' house, and I worked there for nearly three years while studying for my hairdressing qualifications. It was a brutal professional environment, because of the hours and the dynamic of so many women working side by side, and by the time I finally passed my exams I realised that I didn't want to work as a hairdresser at all. But I still didn't have any clear idea of what I'd like to do instead, and one thing I really wish is that I'd had more of an idea of the almost limitless opportunities out there. If you're 16 and leaving school, I want you to know that there are more options than just beauty and hairdressing.

When it came down to it, as a teenager and in my early twenties, all I really cared about was my friends. Growing up, I would be playing out every night and constantly social-ising, and then as soon as I was allowed, I'd be sleeping over at friends' houses every single weekend (getting up to no good, of course. Even though I respected my parents, I was still a teenager after all!). As a younger woman, I hung out in a massive crowd – on Friday nights and the weekends, we would always be together. Sometimes I think those were the best times of my life, because there was no social media and everything just happened in the moment. I must have been about fifteen when the first Nokia smartphone came out, but before that, unless someone had a disposable camera with them, the only memories were the ones you had in your head – at least if you hadn't drunk too much! I look back and feel so grateful that I was part of a generation that didn't have to be so self-conscious about everything; I wasn't endlessly scrolling in my bedroom, comparing myself to other girls. I do think it was easier to be a teenager back then.

I can remember getting male attention from a really young age – I'd probably say an inappropriately young age. Right from the beginning it made me feel massively uncomfortable. I was such an innocent teenager and I certainly didn't have much savvy or confidence in either myself or my body. Any comments or attention from boys made me feel so incredibly shy and totally intimidated me. At the end of school, my year put together an awards ceremony to name each person the 'most likely to be … ' or 'most popular … ', that kind of thing. To my horror, they named me the 'fittest girl' of the year, which I'm sure for a lot of people would have been incredibly flattering, but for me was my actual worst nightmare. I cannot bear being the centre of attention, and that was especially true when I was younger. I found it really hard if I thought anyone was looking at me in a sexual or even romantic way. One of my issues is that I would hate it if anyone thought that *I* thought I was hot, or that I had this big ego. That is so far from who I am. But I also don't like the feeling of having eyes on me, it just makes me want to make myself small.

If you ask any of my friends, my husband or my dad, they'll tell you that I just don't see what other people see when I look in the mirror, and if anyone drew attention to me physically back then, whether it was complimentary or critical, it made me so embarrassed. In my teens and twenties, when I'd get guys asking for my number, or leaving their number under my wipers it never made me think I was attractive. I'd just forget about it and feel like it had happened to someone else, that it wasn't really meant for me. I suppose there was an element of not feeling like I deserved that kind of attention and wanting to deflect anything that might put me in the spotlight.

But unusually for a girl growing up in the noughties, I've never hated my body overall. Of course, I've had insecurities, but I've always known I was slim and the way I look has never been something that I've obsessed over. I've never had an eating disorder or felt any inclination to do anything negative to my body. With the body culture being what it was back then, I was often complimented on being slim, and I definitely had all the benefits that came with having a body that was accepted as 'good'. The only thing I can remember worrying about was my total lack of boobs. At school, comments about girls' bodies were always flying around, and guys would joke about my flat chest, which stuck with me for sure. It was very much the era of big boobs – FHM, Nuts, Page 3 – so even though I was generally happy with my body, I did become really self-conscious about being so flat-chested. The other thing that I became really aware of due to male comments was that I had a prominent thigh gap. Contrary to what you might have seen advertised on Instagram, there is no way to 'get a thigh gap'; it's something that is anatomically determined by the bone structure you're born with. I can remember boys talking about it in a really degrading way, asking me if it was for 'easy access'.

I think I've always been a bit scared by male attention. I know some women like the interest, but I'm the complete opposite – it makes me feel incredibly sensitive. When I was younger, and men would sometimes beep their horns at me, I would be so embarrassed that it actually made me stop going out on my own. Not that it should matter at all, but I've always dressed quite conservatively outside of the gym, so it wasn't like I was even being provocative with my clothing. To this day, I don't feel comfortable walking down the road in my gym kit unless I'm with Romane. If I go to a shopping centre or pop to the store to get something, I always cover myself up with a shirt and jacket and use clothes to make myself look more modest. It's mostly because I often feel really vulnerable whenever a guy I don't know says something about the way I look or looks at me in a certain way for too long. I do think it's sad that I don't feel comfortable wearing what I want outside when I'm on my own, and it certainly shouldn't be that way, but so many of us feel like this and my experiences as a younger woman continue to affect me to this day.

All of this might sound strange considering what I now do for a living – I appreciate the irony that my entire livelihood as a fitness influencer and digital PT is centred on my body and having people notice what I look like. But on social media you are in control of your own content, and the context is very different to being out there in real life. I feel safe in nearly all ways when it comes to my social content. I've also genuinely never experienced that kind of unwanted attention in the gym. It's been a long road for me to get to a point where I'm this comfortable and empowered with my body in the digital space, and I totally understand the number of conflicting emotions that bodies can cause. I also haven't changed in that I still can't bear to be thought of as vain and don't derive much validation from compliments about my body. Let's just say I'm definitely not flexing my biceps in the bathroom mirror each morning thinking how hot I am, or taking 5,000 pouty selfies in the car. But in some ways I have definitely found the confidence to feel comfortable in my own body, and that has come to be what I personally think of as sexy – it's one of the reasons that when I first set up my community I called it Strong & Sxy (it's now the STRNG app).

My journey to finding this acceptance hasn't been a straight road, and while I would love to say that I did everything for the right reasons, that wouldn't be entirely true. I recently found the paperwork from when I originally signed up to the gym, and it reminded me what prompted me to go in the first place. I'd been walking my dog through a field, and as I passed by a group of lads, they started making this noise like a ball bouncing up and down and I remember thinking, 'Oh my God, they think my bum looks fat or something, I'd better go to the gym'. Looking back, this was totally ridiculous as I was so slim, but I thought about that encounter for a long time after it had happened. The sad reality is that I didn't start going to the gym to improve my own fitness or to make my figure look a certain way for myself. It was because of what a bunch of boys I'd never met had randomly shouted one day as I was walking my dog.

I was coming up to twenty-one and I'd been in the same relationship since my late teens. I didn't feel great about myself in any way, and I wasn't feeling fulfilled by my relationship – exactly the opposite, in fact. My work was solid, but not inspiring or interesting, and I felt quite down. I wouldn't say I was technically depressed; it was more that there wasn't that much colour or excitement in my life outside the love of my friends and family. It wasn't that there was anything badly wrong, although looking back I was definitely absolutely miserable sometimes; it was more that nothing really felt right. I didn't have any passion or fire for anything other than being with my friends. In fact, it was one of my best friends, Aimee, who got me into doing fitness classes at the gym because she had been going for a while and had made it sound fun; I would never have had the balls to go on my own.

After the first few times I was totally and utterly hooked. All the classes were aerobic-based, but I also did body pump, which would set the foundations for weightlifting later on. I did a spin and body pump class on Wednesdays and Fridays, then legs, bums and tums on a Thursday. I found it so addictive, and before I knew it I had built a proper routine, which was probably my first step to creating some discipline in my life. I can remember that very first class – being taught how to do a squat, and moving my body in ways I never had before. I was in serious agony the next day, and can still almost feel how much it hurt; I couldn't sit on the toilet or walk down the stairs because my legs were so, so tight. The classes were run by a husband-and-wife team, and they made me feel immediately comfortable, so when Aimee stopped going, I carried on. It wasn't just the endorphins that got me into it, it was because it gave me structure and something to look forward to through the week. Five years later I was still going to every class religiously.

When I started the classes I was quite skinny, without any curves to speak of. I weighed 8 stone 3lb and had done for years. I can't really remember noticing any changes to my body, but I think that is mainly because I wasn't paying much attention to it. While a negative comment about how I looked had spurred me on to go to the gym in the first place, the reason I continued wasn't because it made me look a certain way or because I had a body goal. I was totally uneducated about how exercise and nutrition could change your body; I didn't know anything about any of the various muscle groups or how to work on a particular part of your physique. Generally, the girls I knew who went to the gym

21

were all focused on losing weight, which I wasn't, so for me it was just the pure entertainment and the way it made me feel inside – happy, safe, and in a place where I could be myself and do something I loved – that kept me coming back every week.

It wasn't until two or three years after starting the classes that I really became aware of how much they had changed the way I looked. I was particularly into the body pump classes, with the steps and Les Mills barbells, and had started challenging myself to push my body further. This will make you laugh, but back then I thought only men could have six packs. I didn't realise that we all had the same muscles, so when I saw my stomach starting to look shredded I was really confused about where my abs had come from. I remember taking a picture (just for myself) of a proper little bicep popping out – there's no doubt that those classes set me on a great course for building my body over the coming years. But I wasn't eating anywhere near enough calories for the work I was doing. Again, this was something that wasn't intentional, I just didn't have the knowledge or experience to understand how to fuel my body properly. I can't remember having a single conversation about protein or macronutrients back then – there wasn't the abundance of information that there is today, and although social media was on the rise, I wasn't following anyone who talked about fitness from a physiological point of view; I just had no point of reference.

I do remember the first time I saw a few of the early fitness girls on Instagram, though, and I just thought, wow. Those girls look amazing, I would love to try to do what they've done. I started thinking about it more and more and over the course of a few weeks began psyching myself up to go into the weight room. Of course, I was completely intimidated – I'd been going to the gym for three years by this point, but the weight room had always felt massively beyond reach, not only because it was a gendered space with a bunch of big lads, but because I thought I would embarrass myself. When I mentioned to my boyfriend that I was thinking of going into the weight room, he just looked at me as if to say, 'Why would you want to do that?' I didn't feel he was being supportive and it knocked my confidence. It took me a long while to get back to a place where I could challenge myself to take that next step.

Thankfully, I did get there in the end, but it's really important to acknowledge that your motivation and ambitions can be derailed by those around you – something I will explore more in the next chapter. When I did finally make it into the weight room, I was pleasantly surprised at how my fitness classes had laid the groundwork for weight training. From my form – how to squat and hold your core in place – to knowing the value of consistency, those five years had absolutely given me a head start. Of course, I was still too nervous to go alone, but luckily I had the support of two friends, Emma and Chiara, who were also interested in trying the weight room. The first time was on a Saturday afternoon, and the gym in our little leisure centre was completely dead. I can remember just going around all the machines and trying them out, having literally no idea what each one was for. All three of us were just getting on each of the machines and trying to read the instructions without a single clue what we were doing. It all felt so brand new, and such an amazing challenge, I couldn't wait to get properly stuck in.

Very quickly I built a routine in the weight room and left my fitness classes behind. My friends both dropped off, but it was ok because by that point I'd already become more comfortable with being there on my own. It only takes a few times before that initial dread fades and before you know it things that felt so unachievable and daunting become natural and normal. I always say to anyone who is intimidated by the gym that I know exactly how they feel, and my advice is to start with a friend, even if it's just a few times, as it will make it easier for you to contemplate going on your own – you just have to make it over that first and highest hurdle.

I ended up befriending a couple of guys who were really into their training (I know, it was very out of character, but they were so good to me), and they taught me all about the different muscle groups and which machines worked which ones. While weightlifting and weight rooms can look massively bro-like, and girls may feel like they will be judged for the amount they are lifting or their technique, I've actually found the community to be hugely supportive. These guys might look big and unapproachable, but more often than not you'll find them to be really warm and helpful, though of course every gym has its own vibe and some are more friendly than others. I didn't have a personal trainer, and for a year until I met my husband it was just me teaching and guiding myself, building my body in a totally random way. That was the start of my weightlifting story, and it's one which has completely and utterly changed my life for the better.

Obviously, weightlifting remains very gendered and there's a lot of misinformation out there. I think one of the biggest issues when you boil it down is that so many women think weightlifting will make them look less attractive to men. Sex appeal is so subjective, and what people deem to be sexy or what is seen as an asset – a big bum, big boobs, no boobs or a tiny waist – changes from decade to decade. In the 1950s it was all about curves, and the 1990s was all about being stick thin. When I was young in the noughties, it was all about being super-skinny, size zero or just having massive, often fake boobs. Thankfully, these days there is more of a movement towards a strong female body as the ideal, and the Kardashian-like curvy look is back in.

Not everyone agrees with what is attractive, and social media is a space where you will be criticised from every angle. Sometimes people will criticise you in two entirely contradictory ways even in the same comment. The reality is that these are just opinions, and opinions are coloured by people's own life experiences and insecurities. I'm really lucky that I generally have a positive community who support me, but with nearly 2.5 million people watching what I do, of course I get some hate here and there. I find that with negative body comments, it goes in phases with periods of criticism followed by periods of quiet, and most often the comments come from people that don't follow me, but who might have seen a video or picture on their explore page and then click through to leave a negative comment before going on their way. I always wonder how many other people's posts they comment on to make themselves feel good. Do they feel better after posting ten negative comments in a row? Or twenty perhaps?

The comments are usually focused on me looking 'too manly', and my muscles get a lot of heat, especially my thighs. Apparently, I don't look feminine enough, and my body doesn't look the way a woman's 'should'. Often, I get people accusing me of taking steroids, which is crazy, because I'm a tiny person in real life. I'm not being funny; if I was taking steroids I'd be wanting my money back, because they are definitely not working! I've reached a place now where I can take it as a compliment – if people think I'm taking steroids, it must mean they think I have impressive muscles, so I'll take that. If people don't believe that I've achieved this through nutrition and training, that's their problem. On the flip side, I also get comments saying I'm too skinny and I need to eat a burger. The truth is that, as a woman, your body is never going to please everyone and there will always be someone out there who wants to put you down or make themselves feel better by trying to push your buttons. I do find it strange, though, that people unleash such a horrible side of themselves online – they wouldn't cross the road to say the same thing to my face on the street, so why do they feel they can do it in my DMs? Ultimately, it's the same thing.

When you see men making negative comments about a woman's body being strong, you have to wonder what it is that triggers them. Does it threaten or intimidate them? Of course, my body might not be what they find attract-ive – that's totally fine, because we all have our own tastes.

But why put someone down over their body? I know my husband finds me attractive, so I don't really care what any other man thinks, but it is interesting this obsession with certain body measurements being acceptable for females and others apparently falling foul of the 'standards'. No woman has to conform to a certain body type or body shape beyond the one she personally finds attractive and comfortable. Femininity isn't a body type – you can be feminine and slight, feminine and voluptuous, feminine and strong.

As for how these comments impact me, I can't say I've ever really worried about looking masculine. Instead, I've always felt proud about being a role model for strong women. Part of that is because I have my husband's support in everything I do, and with his background in fitness and bodybuilding, I know that he sees my shape as something to be proud of rather than to slate. We also have such an incredible community around us who just have no time for that kind of negativity. And here's the thing: I like the way my muscles look. I like looking strong, and even more, I like feeling strong. That is what makes me feel my most attractive, and while I would never call myself sexy, I am definitely at my most confident. I have never let the negative comments make me think, 'Oh God, I shouldn't train my quads', or anything like that. Training has changed my outlook on almost everything. These days, a group of lads laughing about my bum could still make me feel vulnerable, but it wouldn't make me want to change how I look. I'm happy in myself, I love what I do and I'm so proud of what I've achieved, so I would never let a few shitty comments undermine that.

There is, of course, still a pressure to stay slim and for many women, fitness is still about losing weight; I know a lot of women still struggle with thinking that lifting weights is going to make them look manly and bulky, and that men won't find them attractive because of that. Of course, there are women out there who do want to look bulky and that is their goal with weightlifting and that's great for them. But the reality is, if you're lifting weights and simply eating normal food, you're not going to suddenly bulk up. That is *hard work*. The female body doesn't have the level of testosterone required to just start piling on muscle overnight – it's hard enough for men to build, let alone us. This fear of weights and lifting is something that needs to be addressed because so many women are missing out on one of the best ways to improve their strength, stamina and fitness, all because they have this misguided idea that dumbbells are going to turn them into the Incredible Hulk. No way is that happening! It's super-hard for females to build muscles naturally, and it would take years of increased calories and lifting weights to get there.

I think because of how I look – because I'm slender and toned even with the muscle mass – it's shown lots of my followers that they can build a strong femininity with weights and create lean muscle rather than coming out looking like Arnie. Strength training can help with weight loss, but it also builds muscle and bone mass at the same time. For women it's especially beneficial because it guards against osteoporosis and age-related muscle loss, with the added advantage of strengthening your ligaments and tendons to prevent you from injuring yourself. So, the fact that only 24 per cent of British women meet the government guidelines for strength training (twice weekly) is a real missed opportunity and it's something that is hurting women's health.

As for the comments, it's not just the hateful ones that I've had to learn to navigate, but the degrading ones too, which make you feel totally sexualised. I know there are people out there who would say, well, you're on Instagram showing your body in tight clothes, what do you expect? I always respond by underlining that I showcase athletic training, and that just like in real life, a woman shouldn't have to wear a sack to protect herself from unsolicited sexual advances. It's sad that we haven't moved on from the narrative that what a woman wears can legitimise sexual abuse and intimidation. When I first started out on Instagram, for the first couple of years I had a lot of men following me – I think the demographic was about 50/50 – and I could never understand it because I didn't post anything even slightly provocative. I used to hate it so much, not because I wouldn't want a man to try some of the techniques I use – I want to inspire men as much as women to make a positive change to their life – but because of the kind of comments and messages I received from them. Let's just say they weren't particularly interested in my lifting technique. The suggestive, sexual comments were one thing, the creepy messages and unwanted images another, and I just didn't want to read any of them. And seeing those comments isn't just potentially harmful for me, but for all the women following me too; they just serve to re-enforce the idea that a woman's worth is tied to how sexy men find her.

As soon as I started posting my workout videos, the amount of women following me shot up, so these days it's a much smaller ratio of men, which I definitely prefer. The reality is that as a woman you are going to be subject to all kinds of outside influences on how you feel about yourself and your body. There will be comments, both positive and negative, online or offline, which can shape your view of what a 'good' body and a 'bad' body looks like. Whether you only have a few followers or thousands, whether you're in school or on the street running for the bus, whether it's your dad or your boyfriend or your sister or best friend – without even realising it, you will take on and internalise a lot of these opinions (and I say opinions because that's all they are, and what's more they're constantly changing) and they will have the power to make you feel confident or insecure, which can have a massive impact on your life. It starts as soon as you become a teenager, and navigating it and avoiding letting the worst of it affect you is super-important for your happiness both as a young woman and for the future.

When I was younger, I was so embarrassed to even be noticed, and was really affected by the things boys and men said to me, whether it was being flat-chested, having a big bum or a thigh gap. I still sometimes feel sensitive about showing my body in public, but through my training I have reached a point where those types of comment no longer have the power to make me feel negative about myself. Sure, I can still feel scared by the attention sometimes, but now I have so much strength behind me, even that has lessened. There would have been times when I was younger that I might have looked at my body and felt there was something wrong with it, that perhaps it wasn't feminine enough, because of all the standards and expectations I'd taken in. Now I realise what utter crap that is. So much of finding your body confidence as a woman is shedding these attitudes and building a whole new framework for yourself in terms of what makes you feel good and what you feel looks good.

Along with that process, you will probably find that you shed other elements of your life too, from relationships to jobs, and build entirely new expectations for yourself. That's what happened to me – all it has taken is a few dumbbells and a lot of hard work and my whole life turned upside down.

STEP ONE RECAP:

- The first step to mental strength is to work on finding something that you love. Whether it's fitness or something else that brings colour to your life, having something to look forward to, that you feel passionate about, is one of the most important things you can do for yourself.
- Focus on your own voice. As a woman, you will be bombarded with messages about how you should feel about yourself, and that is particularly intense when it comes to your looks and body. With so many different opinions out there and attitudes changing so often, it doesn't make sense to listen to any of them.
- The only body shape worth coveting is the one that makes you feel strong and confident. Forget about looking too manly or too curvy – or too anything.
- It's not unusual to feel intimidated by sexual attention, even as a more mature woman. Abuse of any kind should never be tolerated, whether online or off. While it remains a sad fact of life, remember that you don't ever deserve it.

- Fitness can help build a routine and bring discipline to your life. Achieving your goals makes you feel proud of yourself, and that in turn raises your self-esteem and confidence.
- Sexy is something you feel from within and isn't something you can get to through validation from others, so focus on making yourself happy first because everything else follows from that.

I'm handing over to my glamorous husband Romane now for the first step to physical strength, an A–Z of muscles.

STEP ONE TO PHYSICAL STRENGTH: HOW MUSCLE IS MADE

What is muscle anyway?

Romane

Hello to everyone reading! Congratulations on taking this first step towards building strength! I know how hard it is from personal experience, but you will be absolutely amazed by what you can achieve, both physically and mentally, from lifting weights. Life-changing is an understatement. Today, reading this, you might think the idea of getting from where you are now to the body and mindset you'd like to accomplish is too steep a climb, but I can tell you, if you take things one step at a time, set short-term goals and focus on what is directly in front of you, it's 100 per cent achievable.

So, let's start at the very beginning. When it comes to the physical side of things, when we talk about strength, what people usually think of is the size of your muscles. It's important to say now that there is often a difference between the perception of strength vs actual strength. If you are at a low level of body fat, your muscles will look more defined ('ripped', 'shredded'), whereas if you're carrying more body fat, your muscular structure will be less visible. That totally does not mean you are less strong – in fact, often the opposite is true. Additionally, you will find there are people that can lift incredibly heavy weights without looking anywhere near as 'big' as you would expect, because they have trained their body to contract their muscles better. While the way your body looks can have an impact on your confidence and can be an awesome result of your hard work, strength is about so much more than how you look. As a professional bodybuilder, I understand the aesthetics of strength and building muscle better than most, but still, hand on heart, the aspect I love the most about living strong is the way it makes you feel.

But let's get down to brass tacks. Unless you've been revising for your GCSE Biology recently, how you build muscle might be a bit of a mystery – don't worry, this isn't a test, but having a bit of an idea of what is actually physiologically happening in your body can really help you visualise building your muscles as you exercise. The body is made up of different kinds of muscles, like the heart muscle for example, but for the purposes of this book we'll be focusing on skeletal muscle. Made from myofibrils (the long proteins which make the basic thread-like structure of the muscle), there are 650 different skeletal muscles in the body (one for the pub quiz!). Each of those muscles has the ability to contract when it receives a message from the brain via your nervous system. The better your muscles are at reacting to those messages, the better they will contract – practice definitely makes perfect. Over time, you will find certain moves become easier to make, simply because your body has become more efficient and effective at communicating with the muscles due to consistent repetition and a stronger mental focus on creating certain movements (known as the mind to muscle connection).

At the same time, of course, you will be building muscle mass. The way you grow your muscles – known as hypertrophy – is by breaking the threads of the muscle tissue through applying a stress greater than it had previously been adapted to. This muscular damage is why you're so sore a day or two after a workout (often known as DOMS or Delayed Onset Muscle Soreness). As the muscle repairs, the fibres will increase in size to respond to the additional pressure, and over time this will grow the size of your muscles. This process, like everything in your body, is dictated by your individual DNA, which is why some people will build muscle incredibly quickly – the 'genetic freaks' – while others will be 'hard gainers'. Most people will be somewhere in the middle, but it is important to remember that there is nothing you can do to change your genetic advantage here and it really can be significant. If things seem to be going slowly for you, absolutely know that it's not because you're doing anything wrong, we all just progress at a different pace.

The kinds of exercises Lisa and I do in the gym work by progressively pushing the muscles to adapt to heavier and heavier weights, prompting the body to tear and repair the muscle tissue time and time again. It's really that basic.

During the first six months to a year of lifting you will make the most improvement. This is because your muscles are almost in shock and will respond very quickly to the additional pressure you are putting on them. Everyone has their own unique, natural limitations on how strong they can get, and you can reach somewhere around that threshold pretty quickly without too much time and focus on diet and training. You could train four or five times a week and make huge initial progress within your first year of lifting, until your body hits those barriers, then things get much harder and you start looking at minimal year-on-year gains and progress requiring focused diet and training. By this point, you are having to push your body past its boundaries, which is why it takes so much longer from here on out.

As you gain more experience, you are also able to build your mind to muscle connection. Many people will just lift, pulling or pushing the weight from A to B without thinking intentionally about the muscles that are being used. But the more you can improve the mind to muscle connection, the better the contraction you will get on that muscle. It takes a lot of time to develop this form, and only when you're entering more advanced stages will you be able to really master a great contraction.

Another major factor in muscle growth is the role of hormones. When you talk about muscles and hormones, most people's thoughts immediately go to testosterone and there's a good reason for that. The vast majority of the testosterone in both men and women (yes, women – the ovaries produce both oestrogen and a small amount of testosterone) is bound in the body. But around 2 per cent is free to get involved with muscle growth, increasing the rate of protein synthesis (the process by which different proteins join together to make muscle fibres, known as an *anabolic* pathway) and making the muscle cells more sensitive to free testosterone. What's more, weightlifting itself can increase the amount of testosterone produced, meaning the more muscle you build, the more of the hormone is created to help you keep gaining.

Anabolic steroids, which you will probably have also heard about in connection with weightlifting (more on this later in the supplements chapter), basically mimic the function of testosterone and therefore facilitate muscle growth. There are many issues with steroid misuse, which we will address later, but that's essentially why people take them. However, you still need to train and tear and repair your muscles no matter what – there is no supplement that you can take that will suddenly just make you muscular in your sleep.

All of this takes time. You cannot build muscle overnight, because it is incredibly hard work for your body to build tissue this way. That is one of the reasons it is so misguided for women to be nervous of building muscle too quickly. That just will not happen, and even if it did, the rate at which you lose muscle is so rapid that it would be a temporary and reversible situation.

It's worth mentioning here the differences between the sexes in terms of building muscle. Except in rare cases, men have more testosterone than women and can therefore build more muscle at a faster rate. This is on a massively sliding scale, however. Those men with a genetic advantage will have the ability to build muscle mass insanely quickly and their potential for growth will be huge. Others who are hard gainers will struggle to reach 5 per cent of that mass. The same goes for women. It certainly isn't the case that men can build more muscle because they are tougher or more dedicated. It's just chemistry, simple as that. A trans man who uses testosterone supplements may find he is more able to build muscle, whereas a trans woman using testosterone inhibitors may find it far harder to build muscle than she did before she started medication. Women can expect to gain about three or four pounds of muscle tissue in their first year of weight training, whereas men can expect about double that, but of course that is an average. Following that first year, men might add two pounds a year, while for women it could be a pound or even less. Gaining muscle is absolutely a marathon, not a sprint.

While we're on the subject of genetics – you can build and lose any muscle in your body, but you can't reposition it or completely change its shape. That is genetically determined, like the length of your bones or the colour of your eyes. This is something which I feel needs to be addressed far more clearly by the fitness industry and especially by the fitness community online. One of the best examples is the ab muscles. We have all seen images of perfectly symmetrical six- or eight-packs, but for the vast majority of people, their stomach, no matter how much they train, will never look like that. The length of your muscles and where they attach to the bone isn't something you can change. Say you have genetically short biceps with a 'flat' muscle – you will never get an Arnie arm, no matter how hard you hit the gym. As a bodybuilder I'm super-aware of this truth, but many people who are new to the gym believe that if they lift weights they will eventually look exactly the same as someone they follow on the 'gram. Instead, it's so much better to understand that all you can impact is the size of a muscle, and your ambition should be to make the most of your heredity rather than fight against it. Comparison is a massive evil when it comes to weightlifting, and there are so many people online who say that if you work out like them, you will look like them. It's just not true and it leads so many people to have false expectations.

I mentioned it a bit earlier on, but it's definitely important to also understand how body fat comes into play. Again, this is another genetically determined relationship as you cannot choose where on your body your fat is held. Due to evolution (you can't fight that shit!), women generally store a much higher percentage of body fat than men, in preparation for fertility and lactation, and oestrogen levels are thought to be key in how much each individual will be keeping on tap. For men, it's actually low levels of testosterone that leads to a bigger belly – which is why, as men age, you'll often see a pot belly developing. Some people naturally store their fat in their bum and thighs rather than across their stomachs, which means they can run at a fairly high percentage body fat but still have visible abs. Obviously, if the opposite is true, you could be at a really low level of body fat and still not have defined stomach muscles, even though you have done all the training and more. I absolutely don't want to say that you can't change your body to an insane level and work towards the very best version of yourself, but there are some things you just cannot alter. Anyone who tells you differently is simply lying and trying to make money from you.

We touched above on the degradation of muscle (known as muscle atrophy) and how damn quickly that can happen. You can spend three years training consistently, fuelling your body with the perfect nutrition and build an amazing muscle mass. Then, because of injury or a need to pause your training, your muscle mass will start to deteriorate within four weeks. It's literally a case of use it or lose it. Our bodies are incredibly and impressively adaptive. If you tell your body you only need your muscles to walk to the fridge and open it a few times a day, that's all it will believe it needs to do. It's not like the muscle cells disappear, but when they're damaged, your body doesn't bother repairing them, meaning over time the fibres get smaller and smaller.

If you trained for two months and gained two pounds of muscle mass, two months out of the gym will see you losing nearly all of that muscle mass.

But what about muscle memory? Well, any previous training definitely helps you rebuild muscle quicker when you return to the gym after time away. This is because your nervous system has already been trained in how to lift a certain weight, so the pathway is already established – the memory is in your brain, not in the actual muscle. And unless you have been entirely sedentary for a very long time, there will still be a small amount of muscle present (it can take years to totally lose all of your muscle mass, depending on how much you had built), and that means you start from a higher point than when you began at zero.

Another way you lose muscle mass is when you put your body into starvation mode. If you don't consume enough calories, along with the body fat that is burned to keep your body going, you will also catabolise (consume for energy) your muscles too. The body will reduce your muscles down to the bare minimum it needs to function before it goes full throttle into the body fat. This is the big reason why we absolutely do not recommend any kind of starvation or crash diet: you do not create strength by starving yourself – in fact, it's the complete opposite. It is also why you have to be conscious of your cardiovascular training when you are looking to build muscle. Now I'm not saying that cardio isn't great for your health; it is absolutely vital to your fitness levels, which will have a huge impact on your overall strength. But if you burn all of your calories through long-distance running or high-intensity cardio, you will have a lower level of energy available for muscle building and repair, and if your net calories run too low, your body might start catabolising your muscles for fuel to run your body. In that context, the body can neither build nor maintain muscle mass.

What is less spoken about is how incredible weightlifting is for the cardiovascular system. Lifting weights for an hour a week has been shown to reduce the chance of having a heart attack or stroke by up to 70 per cent – weights give your heart and cardio system an insane workout in their own right. There's even research that suggests weightlifting is *better* for guarding against heart disease than cardio. It's definitely time to ditch this idea that weightlifting is just for bulking, whereas cardio is for your heart and general health – the two are far more connected than we have been led to believe. This is another reason why I think it's so important to confront the gendered stereotypes around weightlifting, because they discourage so many women from getting into the weight room and that is massive for their future heart health.

So now you have a bit of a grounding in what's going on in your body when you build muscle, you might be thinking, 'Great! I'm ready to go!'. But then you get to the gym, walk over to the weightlifting equipment and suddenly you feel completely intimidated and have no idea where to start. Perhaps you end up turning away and pretending you were walking to the water fountain. Well, stop right there, because as daunting as those machines can look if you've never used them before, they are usually very straightforward.

Before you go to the weight room, it's worth learning a little bit about your muscle groups and the types of exercise that target each of them. Lisa and I will often work around the push-pull-leg split, dividing the body into three sections where each is trained separately. The push literally trains the upper body muscles you use to push; the pull the upper body muscles used to pull; and well, the legs is self-explanatory. As you focus on each area in different sessions, it means the other areas can recover and repair while you're still building elsewhere, but it also ensures there's not too much time in between workouts, so you're keeping the consistency needed to persuade your body not to catabolise any muscle tissue you have built. You'll hear the word consistency a lot when it comes to strength training, and that's because without it, you just won't progress.

PUSH MUSCLES

Chest, **Shoulders**, **Triceps** (the back of the upper arm, responsible for arm extension)

PULL MUSCLES

Back, **Traps** (trapezius – the diamond-shaped muscle that extends up the back of the neck, down the spine and outward across the shoulders) and **Biceps** (the front of the upper arm, in charge of bending the forearm to the upper arm)

LEGS

Glutes (gluteal muscles, aka your bum), **Quads** (front of thigh), **Hamstrings** (back of thigh) and **Calves**.

It's worth identifying the muscles listed above on your body and thinking a little about how they work and the movements that isolate their function. Then, when it comes to using the machines, each one will have instructions on the side of the machine, so you can literally just read what each one is for and how best to use it. Take the time to really engage with it, adjusting the seat and handles and any other variable before you put any weight on. I would always recommend doing a set or two with a very light weight or even no weight to make sure everything is in the right place

48

for you. And remember, there is no rush – no one is scoring you, and even if you feel like all eyes are on you, try to hold to the truth that everyone is caught up in their own work-out (and let's be honest, themselves), so don't get too flustered.

It's always good to have a plan of how many reps and sets you want to do before you start. Lisa has put together a plan to take you from beginner to more advanced, which you'll find at the back of the book, and our STRNG app will have more information to help you plan your workouts if you need it. The weight you are looking for is the amount that enables you to complete your sets before you totally fatigue. It's a bit of a trial and error process and you might find you set the weight too low or too high at first. That's one of the reasons I really recommend keeping a diary of what you managed to lift and how it felt, so next time you can adjust the weight accordingly.

Start slowly, adding one weight as per the machine instructions, then try the exercise and see how it feels. If it feels very light, add another. The worst mistake you can make is to go in too heavy – though that doesn't mean you shouldn't be looking to progress by adding more weight over time.

With the exercises, you are looking to completely control the movement from A to B. If the weights are crashing up and down, you're wasting your time – you are looking to create tension in a slow, exact movement.

And if in doubt, ask someone! There is zero shame in getting advice when you are trying to master a new skill, especially when it comes to machinery – I mean, you wouldn't expect to just go out and drive without having taken a fair number of lessons, would you? The only danger is in trying to look like you know it all when you don't. If you have a friend who has used the machines before, ask to go with them, or you can always ask the gym instructors or work with a PT – even if it's just for one lesson to get you on track. Getting over that initial embarrassment is so important – and just remember, even I had to use a chest press for the first time ... that was a long time ago now, but we all have to learn, so just dive in and give it a try – you've 100 per cent got this.

STEP TWO TO MENTAL STRENGTH:
YOU ARE THE COMPANY YOU KEEP

Choose your social circle wisely

While I fully believe that both self-confidence and the ability to progress come from within, there is also no doubt in my mind that the people you surround yourself with can have a huge impact on your self-esteem, your expectations for what you can achieve in life and your capacity to find self-fulfilment. Your friends, family, work colleagues and partners all have a big effect on your happiness, and that can influence the trajectory of your life. While you can't choose your family or vet your work colleagues, the other relationships in your life are up to you, so choose carefully.

As a younger woman I was completely oblivious to this and never realised how important the close circle around me was to my own happiness. I had the best parents and brothers, then at school I also had it easy as I made a group of best friends when I was six and we've stayed tight ever since. If anything, the bond I have with them has actually made it harder to make new friends along the way – of course I have lots of acquaintances, but it's hard to compare a new friend with friends you've known your whole life. At school I was really quiet, but I was lucky enough to get on with nearly everybody. So I suppose I took it for granted, having wonderful people around me, because I had never known anything different.

The trouble started after I left school at sixteen. While there had been a few run-ins along the way – I was once targeted by a girl who thought her boyfriend fancied me, and it got so bad that I couldn't to walk to school on my own – generally up to that point I hadn't had any problems with other women. But all that changed when I started my first job as a hairdressing junior. As I was still training, I wasn't actually styling, just washing hair, keeping the salon clean, and bringing clients into the salon then fetching them their teas and coffee. I naively thought that working with so many other girls would result in a really supportive environment, but I soon realised that it was much more complicated. While I got on well with a lot of the women working there, and some of the more mature clients took a particular shine to me, when it came to my colleagues,

I just didn't seem to be able to do anything right. Because I would rather die than disappoint anyone, I always went above and beyond to try to make them happy; I definitely didn't rock the boat, and I was still so shy so it wasn't as if I waltzed in with a big ego. But instead of nurturing me, I felt my inexperience and timid nature were taken advantage of with constant petty put-downs, until I ended up feeling incredibly shitty about myself. To this day I still can't tell you why they seemed to take a dislike to me, but by the time I was about to turn nineteen these experiences made me believe I was the most useless person in the world and that I would never get anywhere. Because it was my first job, I had nothing to compare it to, so everything the boss said about me, I just presumed was true. In the end, even though I qualified and passed my exams, I decided that I didn't have what it took to be a hairdresser – I didn't even particularly enjoy it. I left without ever having the opportunity to use the skills I'd trained so hard to develop.

After that, while still just as lost about what I wanted to do with my life as ever, I soon got another job in the office of a removals company. Once again, I immediately seemed to rub the women working there up the wrong way. One day I had to log in to one of my colleague's computers (at the instruction of my boss) and I found these absolutely horrible emails that had been written about me over the course of several weeks. They weren't based on anything that I'd done, or my performance at the job, it was just nastiness, pure and simple. I can remember going home that night and crying to my mum and she said, 'You're not going back.' It's obviously really hard to get out of a situation like that when you have to earn money to live, but I listened to my mum that time and handed in my notice the very next morning. No one deserves to work in an environment where they feel harassed. Just because it's work, it doesn't mean you have to put up with it.

Back then, I didn't realise that other people could project their insecurities and unhappiness on to me. My family would say things like, 'It's because they're jealous,' but I could never imagine anyone wanting anything I had. I would desperately try to work out what it was about me that had made them hate me so much, and think about how I could change myself to meet their approval. Soon, I just began to expect that women wouldn't like me no matter where I went or what I did. Whenever I met new people, I would have that sinking feeling and look for hints that they had taken against me. My self-talk had become really toxic, and it made me withdraw even further in social situations. People had always taken the mick out of how quiet my voice was, but by this point I sometimes felt I could barely whisper. When you're so young and unsure of yourself, it's impossible to imagine that the way people treat you could have anything to do with them. You just take it all on yourself and presume you're the one at fault. But I was never to blame for the bullying. I'm sure those women made me unhappy and small in a bid to make themselves feel happier and bigger, and I hadn't learned enough about the world to see what was going on. I hadn't realised that it was my job to protect myself from that type of environment and to carve out a place of work that was supportive and positive. Perhaps that's why I've ended up working for myself! But being unhappy with your job because of the people you work with is something that needs to be fixed, whether you make a complaint or explore new professional avenues – don't ever feel like it's not important because it can have a really big impact on you, even if you don't realise it at the time.

I then moved on to work for an electrical utility company. The job itself wasn't the most interesting – I worked as a data analyst, looking at meter readings to determine where engineers were needed. It was a very specific, one-person job, which had to be done the exact same way, in the exact same order, every day. I know that kind of routine might sound a bit mundane, but the people who worked there were so great, and it was so refreshing to not be worrying about work in the way I had become used to. I became really good friends with the girl I sat next to, which was unusual for me because I am so guarded. My next job was at Network Rail, where I was in a team of mostly men, and I found that environment much easier as it reminded me of growing up around my two brothers.

I feel lucky in some ways, because however difficult my work was, I always used to see it as 'just a job' – mainly because I wasn't passionate about it, which I suppose wasn't ideal. But it did allow me to compartmentalise it, and my life outside of work with my friends was always something totally separate. While I would feel really down when people were horrible to me in the office, and of course those feelings would follow me home from time to time, it wasn't as if it ruined my whole life. With my friends and family, I was still happy and upbeat and just the same Lisa as before – always laughing and doing ridiculous, silly things. It was more that those experiences planted a seed, which grew and grew into a serious lack of self-belief.

The backdrop to all of this, and the thing that made it all so much harder to deal with, was another unhappy relationship, one that consumed too much of my life. No matter what choices I made or achievements I got under my belt, this relationship served only to confirm my belief that I was worthless. I met my first boyfriend in my late teens and we were together until I was in my mid-twenties, by which point we were engaged. It was a really long time to be in a relationship with someone and to feel undermined, and it's scary how quickly that can happen.

While I don't judge anyone, I'm just not a one-night stand girl and I have only ever been in monogamous, long-lasting intimate relationships, which I guess comes from my parents, who have been together for so long. When I met my boyfriend, I was so sure that he was going to be the person I would spend the rest of my life with. Looking back, some of it was my fault. I should have walked away right at the start. But I was young and innocent, and he was older than me. We did get on with each other so well, after all. Then, as I got deeper and deeper into the relationship, his family became my family. Years passed and I got used to swallowing all the hurt out of fear of losing my entire life, which I'd built around him. I'd think, 'I'll just carry on because who else is going to want to be with me anyway? I'm not that good, am I? I'm not worth much, so I might as well just stick with him.'

When we bought a flat together, I didn't think twice. He was my life partner and I'd really made my bed now, as we were bound by money, contracts and an engagement ring. I felt we had to become engaged and get married. I didn't feel able to say no. Back then, I didn't have the strength to do what needed to be done. I still hate arguments and any kind of confrontation, and that means that sometimes I just go along with things, even when I know they're bad for me. I was letting life happen to me instead of guiding my own ship and making my own choices, but a lot of that was because I didn't trust my own judgement and felt that I had nothing to offer. I also knew that I would struggle to cope with the sadness and upset, even though I was so unhappy most of the time anyway. The relationship had become such a vicious circle.

On one occasion we were due to go on holiday with a group of my friends and their partners, but a couple of days before we were due to leave he told me he wouldn't be coming as he wanted to go away with his friends instead – meaning I had to go on a couples' holiday with my mates all on my own. I don't remember ever feeling that anything I did was encouraged; I don't remember him ever complimenting me or wanting to spend any time with me. In retrospect, sometimes that was a positive thing because a lot of my social life happened without him as he'd never come to a festival or party with my friends and me. But at the time, I just felt I wasn't interesting enough or important enough for him.

When I look back now, he probably had his own issues and fears and insecurities. We all do. I can only describe my feelings during that time. All my friends and family would say that they loved him, but they didn't love us together. It doesn't matter what anyone else says or thinks, because it's you who has to dig deep to find the strength to make a change for yourself.

My parents have always been very impartial, and believed we needed to make our own mistakes. They were never going to tell me to finish with him, even though sometimes they were concerned for me. There was one instance when I was out shopping with my mum, and he would call me every three or four minutes. I was supposed to be spending time with my mum, so I didn't pick up, but as the calls kept coming through I became more and more anxious. I remember mum voicing her concern. Another time, I'd just passed my driving test and was out practising when the calls started. I knew it was him, and I also knew that I shouldn't pick up, but after eight or nine calls I did pick up – and ended up being pulled over by the police and fined with points on my licence. I was so worried about things flaring up between us that I answered the phone while I was driving: I was that bad. Still, my parents left me to it, because they were wise enough to know they had to let it play out.

I've since seen other friends in a similar situation and have tried to guide them, but while it's easy for others to talk about, it is something you can only do when you're ready. There were a couple of people that I turned to for advice, though – a girlfriend my own age and one of my mum's friends – who both offered me so much support and gave me some perspective. And while I know it's not everyone's cup of tea, I was so unhappy that I also went to see a medium to try to see a way forward. It was actually my mum's suggestion and I was really sceptical at the time and didn't really feel that it was a good idea, but what did I have to lose when I was already at rock bottom? I remember taking my engagement ring off so he wouldn't know that I was in a relationship and as I would never do anything on my own, of course I brought a friend with me. I've kept the DVD of the session and it is truly uncanny. The first thing he said was that I was going to get really stuck into fitness and move into the industry, working for myself. At the time, the idea that I would have my own fitness company and would be self-employed wasn't just unlikely, it was laughable! I was an analyst in an office working for Network Rail; I hardly knew anyone who worked for themselves, let alone had any aspirations to do it myself. I was just sitting there looking at him thinking, 'This is such crap', but me being me, I still went along with it. He then said that I was going to meet my dream man – tall and dark and who would also be in fitness – and we would live in a massive house with a huge kitchen and a nice car. He also said that I was going to move overseas, another thing I would never have dreamed I'd do. I'm not sure I actually believe he could see into the future (though it was extremely good guesswork!), but I do think the reading planted a seed in my mind. The fact that I have my own business is still a shock to me now, but back then the idea seemed crazy. And moving overseas? Are you joking? I'm such a home girl and I love my family so much. Yet looking back now, it taught me that you can never predict the road your life is going to go down.

I had met my ex when I was so young, and we were both part of the bigger network in our town. I was in my late teens when I fell for him – there are always those boys who are a bit older and drive their own cars and back then he was exactly the kind of person I thought I should be with. But everyone could see that it wasn't right. With my fitness, I don't remember him ever commenting on anything about my body over the five years I was going to classes. If he could see that I was finding confidence from my progress he didn't say anything about it and he didn't seem to notice any of the changes that my body went through.

What was it that gave me the strength I needed? I still ask myself that question. The year we split we had gone on holiday together to Thailand for two weeks, and I can remember how deflated I was when we came back, because I really hadn't had a good time. I was then set to go off on a girls' trip to Ibiza. My friend Nadine had just split with her long-term boyfriend and we were going to take her mind off things – to dance, to have a laugh and just forget about everything. On one of the first days, she started talking to a group of lads and we all just fell into hanging out for the rest of the holiday. I think it was seeing my friend blossom again after having had such a hard time that set the wheels in motion for me. We were only there for five days, but I suddenly realised I deserved so much more. Here was Nadine with her confidence growing, taking her next step forward, and I just thought it could be me too. It was long overdue.

When I got back, I mustered up the courage to talk frankly to my ex and we ended our relationship. Again I can't put my finger on where I found the strength from, but something had just clicked. I hadn't changed overnight – I was still the girl who didn't know how to say no – but there was just this sense that it was now or never going around in my head. Ibiza had been a massive wake-up call and I just knew I needed to change things.

I do think he could understand why it wasn't working for us. The memory of the break-up still haunts me even to this day, but as soon as it was over, I felt like a massive weight had been lifted off my shoulders. Suddenly I was free and could do whatever I wanted to. I can't even describe the relief and elation – it was like my life had started all over again.

Most people would probably want to go a bit wild at this point – to go out partying, knock back a few drinks and kiss some boys – but my first and only thought was to get to that weight room and see how far I could push myself and my body. After that, I made up my mind to always do what I wanted to, and never let anyone, especially the man that was supposed to love and support me, stop me from achieving my goals.

As a sidenote and a little reminder of how destiny sometimes comes into play, if Nadine hadn't broken up with her boyfriend and gone to Ibiza, I would never have started my Instagram or met my husband or had the life that I do today. Basically, Nadine stayed in touch with the guy she'd been chatting to on holiday, and he came to visit her in London with some of his friends, and she asked me to come along too. That night I got chatting to his friends, and as I was telling one of them about my classes and going to the weight room, he suggested that I start an Instagram account to chart my journey. He then proceeded to pull out his phone and show me some amazing girls who were sharing short workout videos and little snippets of their routines, as well as progress reports and challenges that they had set themselves. Back then, I didn't follow anyone like that. I hadn't even realised those accounts existed. I immediately said, 'No way, no one would be interested in me working out in the gym!', but he was really persistent and told me that it would inspire and help other women, and that I would get lots of followers and might even get some work out of it. At the time, I couldn't really make head nor tail of what he was talking about. These days of course everyone knows that there is the potential to build a career from a social media platform, but back then it just wasn't common knowledge.

It took me a while to do anything about his advice, as I kept asking myself why anyone would want to follow me. I had a personal Instagram account, but it was just pictures of me and my friends and definitely not focused on images of myself. The idea of taking gym selfies was overwhelming for me, but at the same time, I was getting more and more into the weight room and had really started to see changes in my body. One day I happened to glance in the mirror before I left the house and I realised that my abs were properly shredded. I had never seen my body like that before. I did a little bicep flex in the mirror and took a selfie, and I was like, holy shit! I was actually blown away at what I was seeing, and then felt really proud of what I'd achieved, and I decided to make the Instagram account, just like the guy suggested.

I didn't tell anyone, not a soul. My thinking was that if it worked, great, everyone would find out anyway. And if not, that's fine too – I'll just delete the account and no one will ever know. I uploaded a few gym snaps, then started to post pictures more regularly. Very quickly I got to 700 followers and I remember thinking, 'Wow, what the hell is going on?' Considering my personal account only had about 250 people following it, you can't help thinking who are these 700 people and what do they want from me? How did they even find me?! When I passed the 1,000 follower mark, I messaged the guy who had suggested I start the account and he was so happy for me. Very soon it felt like something was happening and a few of my friends in the area started to see my account and sent me messages asking, 'Is this you, Lisa?' At the beginning, I remember feeling really cringe and replying that, yeah, it was me, but it was no big deal. I didn't want it to come across in the wrong way or for my friends to think I suddenly loved myself. But I also knew that I was inspiring and motivating other girls, and that kept me going no matter how embarrassing it was when people I knew saw my account. My followers would message to say that my account was giving them the confidence to go into the weight room and the mental focus they needed to push themselves further or start specific challenges, and that became a huge motivator for me.

So that was basically how my Instagram started. Sometimes it's not your closest friends who set your life on a different course, it's someone from the outside, and that is a lesson I need to remember: to stay open to new influences and not always be so guarded. Incidentally, the same guy also helped me do something else I had never believed I would be able to: travel on my own. It was one of those things that, before when I was in my previous relationships, I just felt was beyond me, but now I was ready to prove myself and everyone else wrong. So when he asked me to stay with him in Belgium – as a friend – for some reason I said yes! I wanted to push myself out of my comfort zone, and as there was no one to tell me not to do it anymore, I just went for it. In the end, there wasn't anything to it, but I had built it up so much in my mind that it felt like a huge achievement.

Of course, all of this was leading to the most important relationship in my life: meeting my husband Romane. It was just over a year after I had split with my ex and I hadn't dated anyone in between. Firstly, I'm just not much of a dater, and I really felt that the next person I met would be the person I'd settle down with, so I wasn't really into bothering with anything casual. Secondly, I was just so happy on my own. Everyone always asks how Romane and I met, and I always say that if it wasn't for Instagram, we never would have. I was living in Dunstable, he was three hours' drive away in Bristol, and we had no friends in common. Luckily, he slid into my DMs! I think it helped that I wasn't looking for anything and was really focused on myself, because as the saying goes, it always happens when you least expect it.

Right from the outset, there was just something about Romane that felt different. After he messaged me, complimenting me on some of my pictures, we got talking and I soon started to realise he had so much depth. Obviously, I looked at his profile, and as a PT and IFBB (International Federation of Bodybuilding and Fitness) Pro you can see how incredible his body is, but for him it's all about the hard work and motivation rather than looks. A lot of guys in fitness spend hours in front of the mirror, but Romane was just never that guy. I had never dated anyone with a body like Romane's, but appearance isn't the biggest factor for me. Of course you've got to be attracted to someone, but making a connection is about much more than what someone's pecs look like, and I've always found Romane to be attractive no matter whether he's been off season or show ready. He's always amazing to me.

Pretty soon we'd moved on to Facebook (Romane wanted to make sure I was a real person!), and then I gave him my number and we started WhatsApping each other constantly. Before I knew it, we had arranged our first date at a pub in Oxford, halfway between where we both lived. It was 9 October, to be exact, and somehow I was completely at ease. Usually, going on a date with a guy I really liked would have made me so incredibly nervous that I wouldn't have been able to do it. I would have been an absolute state.

But because I had been so happy on my own and had been doing so well in the weight room and enjoying my freedom, I just kind of thought, if he doesn't like me, that's his problem.

We hit it off straight away. It was the most fun evening and we ended up being the last people to leave the restaurant. The staff were basically throwing us out!

We had so much in common and I was so interested in everything that he was doing and how he had got to where he was. I had absolutely no idea about anything to do with bodybuilding or men's physique culture and I found it so intriguing that I couldn't stop asking questions about it. At the time, Romane said he thought I was joking or being sarcastic, but I found everything that he goes through to transform his body so impressive. The connection was just instant and the next week he came to Dunstable to meet my parents. The following week I went to see him compete in a men's physique show in Liverpool, which was a massive eye-opener, then a few days later we got on a plane to Egypt for our first holiday together. Three months later, he proposed to me by the Trevi fountain in Rome. It's such a cliché to say that when you know, you know. If I'm honest, I think you have to have followed the wrong path to know when something really feels right. Since the moment we met I have felt at ease with myself when I'm with Romane and he has been the support structure behind me, building me up as well as providing a cushion to fall back on when things haven't turned out the way I'd hoped. He is an amazing man, who is so driven and so loving, and being around him has inspired me to live a life beyond anything I had ever thought I was capable of.

Romane's background was tougher than mine, in the sense that he was heavily overweight as a child, having been fed up by his nan, and he felt deeply ashamed of his body. When he was thirteen, he decided to do something about his weight and got into training, firstly with little dumbbells at home and then by joining an independent gym. A few years later he saw a poster for a men's physique competition and decided to just go for it. He told me he had absolutely no idea what he was doing, but went along anyway and won. What he didn't realise at the time was that he has an extraordinary physical shape – what you would call an X structure, with a naturally tiny waist and huge shoulders. He didn't have any idea he was built that way until he started training – only a tiny percentage of people would ever be able to train their body and diet down to look like his, but until you start down the road of adding muscle to your body, you would never know the underlying potential was there. Once he realised what a genetic gift he had been given, he decided to dedicate all his efforts towards competing.

Romane's experiences have given him an incredible wealth of knowledge about all aspects of fitness, and especially nutrition. Before we met, I'd enquired into female physique competitions, just because I was so interested, and had spoken to a guy at my gym about them. I told him what I'd been doing and he asked me what I ate. I recounted my daily calorie intake, feeling super-proud that I'd been so good with my chicken and sweet potato, and he just laughed out loud. He said, 'Lisa you're not eating anywhere near enough.' So I had an idea that my diet wasn't optimum for muscle-making, but it wasn't until I met Romane that I really started to learn more about the nutrition side of strength and understood that in order to gain, I needed to increase my calorie intake to fuel my body. At the time I was extremely lean and wasn't carrying any body fat, so there was just nothing to build muscle from. I wasn't putting my body under too much stress, but you do have to be really careful as a woman as your period requires a certain level of body fat to function properly and I just wasn't taking the care I should have been.

Before I met Romane, I'd probably grab a bit of toast for breakfast, a sandwich for lunch and spag bol for dinner, you know the normal kid of thing. I never ate crap and always ate home-cooked food, but I didn't exactly think about the balance of nutrients. As I got into weightlifting, I started to eat more protein, but it still wasn't anywhere near enough. I didn't know how to calculate protein amounts and I guess I was really nervous about seriously increasing my calories. I think we are just conditioned to think that a 'female portion' should look a certain way, but if you want to build muscle, your plate essentially needs to be absolutely massive, whether you're a man or woman.

Aside from learning so much from Romane, he and I have the same ambitions for life and we both love helping other people – but from when we met to where we are today, there was about to be a lot of upheaval, as well as a huge new test of my work ethic and discipline.

STEP TWO RECAP:

- The people around you have a huge impact on your happiness and quality of life. Negativity and toxicity can be catastrophic for your self-esteem and confidence, so it's worth being really honest with yourself about your relationships and whether individuals are supporting you or holding you back.
- Especially when it comes to romantic relationships, putting up with less than you deserve is a one-way ticket to misery. If you can't trust your partner and they aren't there for you through thick and thin, they are not the right person. While it can be really, really challenging to

find the strength to walk away, having that person in your life will always hold you back.

- No one deserves to be bullied or caught up in emotional abuse. Whether this is at home or at work, it stops you from fulfilling your potential. Your priority should be to get out of the situation.

- Seek out relationships with people whose values align with your own. Know what matters most to you and curate your circle to include others who believe in the same things. For me, it's hard work, support and care, kindness and drive, but others will highlight different qualities.

- It's not always your closest friends who open the door to new opportunities and ways to see yourself in a new light. Be open to new influences while at the same time being aware that not everyone has a place in your life (and not everyone has to be your BFF!).

STEP TWO TO PHYSICAL STRENGTH: MAKING THE MOST OF YOUR MACROS

Protein, fats, carbs - and how much should you be eating?

Romane

Now we know how muscle is made, it's time to have a little look at how you can fuel that process through your diet. So many terms are bandied about by fitness influencers online, so you'll no doubt have heard the term 'macronutrients'. It sounds complex, but all it refers to are the three nutrients we need in large quantities to survive: fats, carbohydrates and protein. All the other nutrients – your vitamins and minerals – are known as micronutrients, because as the name suggests, you need less of them.

Over the years, sensational diets have tried to persuade us that each one of these three essential bodybuilding blocks is toxic or evil in some way. In the late 1940s, the low-fat diet became the mainstream trend, with governments around the world pushing the connection between a high-fat diet and high cholesterol, and therefore heart disease. However, there has never been any definitive evidence that for the 'normal' individual (who wasn't high risk for heart conditions) a diet low in fat either prevented heart disease or led to weight loss. Over the past twenty years, the whole 'low-fat diet leading to low body weight' message has been challenged by both scientists and the fitness industry. But the low-fat ideology is what most of us have grown up with and there is a massive hangover from that, with many people only just starting to realise the difference between good and bad fats and how important a moderate level of fat in a diet can be for managing our appetite.

The next biggest trend was the Atkins Diet in the early noughties (the book was one of the top fifty bestselling books *of all time*), which told everyone that carbs were bad. This is where the 'no bread ever' advice comes from, and instead of a low-fat diet, we were told to only eat cheese, butter and eggs. Today's keto dieters follow a similar programme of high-fat, adequate protein, low-carbohydrate nutrition. At the time of writing this, I'd say we are in the protein era, where protein is the wonder macro and absolutely insane consumption is being promoted while the value of carbs and fats remains contested.

But here's the rub: for a balanced, sustainable nutrition plan, which you will be able to stick to forever, you need all three macronutrients in moderation. None of them are toxic; neither bread nor butter is the devil. Not only do these crazy all-or-nothing ideas about food just make no sense, but are in my opinion actually harmful because they lead to an unbalanced diet and unsustainable restrictions, which in turn can lead to control issues around certain foods. However, I'm also not saying that you can just eat whatever you like, go wild on cream cakes and pizza and expect to achieve all of your body goals.

While I'm going to outline my overall approach to macros below, I want to be really clear right from the start that every single person is an individual – what works for one person might not work for another, and I support whatever works for you. If you love a keto diet, for example, and find it helps you to maintain your body composition, you do you. But if you have struggled in the past with keeping to a diet or are looking to build a nutrition plan to specifically support muscle creation and maintenance, keep reading.

As Lisa mentioned earlier, our whole ethos is about empowering you to make your own choices in the gym, and the same goes for your diet – taking responsibility for what you choose to eat is key to not only building your body, but also building the confidence and esteem that comes with achievement. This is your journey. I'm not the food police and I absolutely do not advocate anything extreme or focused towards perfection. While I don't want to cast shade, any plan that is overly prescriptive or tells you that there is only one 'perfect' way to eat should be given a wide berth. While most people would say that our diet is strict, Lisa and I both have days where we eat things that could be seen as nutritionally poor. But because we have such a solid diet plan, those days don't have any impact on our progress. We can only do that because we understand the body's interplay with the nutrients, and that's what I want to share with you.

So, let's start with the macronutrients and the role they each play in your body and its composition. As protein is the macro most associated with muscle growth, we'll explore that one first. Made up of twenty amino acid building blocks, the proteins in the body have loads of uses. Hormones are proteins, bone is made from proteins and we also use protein as an energy source, as just a few examples. Eleven of the amino acids can be made by the body itself, but nine of them need to come via your diet and are known as 'essential amino acids' – without these, your body can't function. It is possible to get all the protein you need from food, however when you are training and looking to build muscle, the increased demands of protein that you need for hyper-trophy mean that it is often way more convenient to take some kind of protein supplement alongside your food sources, otherwise you can find yourself having to eat con-stantly. I'll address the best kinds of protein supplement and what you should be looking for on page 154.

For muscle growth, protein is absolutely vital. Lisa and I eat some protein at every mealtime, every day. Instead of three main meals with snacks in between, we eat six meals, at 7am, 9.30am, midday, then 3pm, 5pm and again at 7pm to keep topping that protein source up. The human body can't store excess protein in the way it can fats and will just excrete any surplus, so it's far better to eat a little pro-tein several times a day rather than going for it all in one evening meal. When you first begin to adjust your diet to create the optimum environment for muscle growth, it can be really helpful to have a rough guide of how much protein (in terms of grams) you need per day. You may find this a massive increase from what you are usually eating, and for women especially it can take a bit of time to get your head around the sheer volume of food you need to consume to support muscle growth. In general, I would say that if you are following Lisa's fitness plan every day, you should feel confident that the increased protein con-tent of your diet is being metabolised by your body. And remember, you have to eat for the body you want, not the one you've currently got.

So, what is the ideal balance? The generally accepted ratio of protein to body weight for optimum muscle growth is between 1 and 1.5g protein per ½ kg (or lb) of weight. Let's say you're a petite woman who weighs 60kg (approximately 130lb) and works out three or four times a week, then I would say you should be aiming for the upper end – around 150g of protein intake per day, and I always say eat a little more to ensure you have a buffer. For those that consume animal products, that looks like two 200g chicken breasts (31g protein per 100g), a salmon fillet (20g per 100g) and two scrambled eggs (15g). For me at double that weight, that's a lot of food – so you can see why supplements are helpful.

For vegans and vegetarians, there are many foods that can provide a great dose of protein, and it is possible to achieve your strength goals following a plant-based diet, but it is much harder to achieve the same results without supplements. Look, there are people out there who could eat grass all day and genetically still have an incredible physique, but for most people, eating a plant-based diet makes muscle growth more challenging. Generally, when someone who is training goes from a meat-based diet to a vegan diet, they lose a lot of muscle mass and become much slimmer. The longer people have been vegan, the better chance they have of building and maintaining muscle, but when you first go from eating meat to becoming a vegan, you will definitely notice a big difference. That's not a knock on vegans at all; there are so many health and environmental reasons to opt for a plant-based diet, but it's just being realistic.

Animal protein is almost a pre-packaged dietary source, offering you all the amino acids you need. A combination of nuts, beans, grains and legumes can achieve the same result, but you'll need to consume about 25 per cent more plant-based proteins for the same benefits, and the issue with that is that both beans and legumes contain a lot more carbohydrate, which will have an impact on fat storage (see page 85).

With protein, timing is critical, another reason why supplements like protein shakes are so useful. You have to remember that even when your body is sleeping, it's breaking down and building protein. Every time you eat a good amount of protein, around 30g, you set off a burst of protein building which lasts about three hours. So if you're only eating protein at lunch or dinner time, for the rest of the day and night (the remaining twenty-one hours) your body will only be able to break down the protein. Training the muscles through weightlifting sets your body up to respond to the protein you feed it, and you have this little window of opportunity before and after your gym session to get your protein in and maximise the impact of your workout. Going back to what we learned in the last chapter, lifting weights (or resistance exercise) breaks down muscle, so you need a fresh, ready and waiting intake of amino acids to repair and increase the size of the myofibrils. If your body runs out of that supply, it won't repair the muscles to the best of its ability, and you won't gain as much muscle as quickly or as easily.

That is why I always recommend eating 20g of protein before or immediately after each workout. For Lisa and me, it's not such an issue, because our diet is structured so that we know there is enough protein in our bodies at all times. But for those who don't have such a solid structure in place, ensuring you have a protein influx pre- and post-workout is one of the easiest and most important things to do from a diet perspective. If you skip breakfast, make sure you get your nutrition in before and after you train. As well as the hit of protein, I also recommend a carb intake at the same time, because that will raise insulin, which in turn slows protein breakdown.

On that note, now you've got your protein nailed, let's have a look at your carbs. Remember when I mentioned that if your body goes into starvation mode, it will turn to muscles to break down the protein for an energy source? Well, the right amount of carbs in your diet will ensure that doesn't happen, and that is vital for both muscle growth and maintenance. Carbohydrates are the main source of energy for the body. When you eat carbs, you give your body energy reserves in the form of glycogen. All glycogen is made up of lots and lots of glucose molecules, and it exists in a triglyceride form (excess glucose molecules which lay down as fat for long-term storage) and simple glycogen (for the short-term energy reserve). You'll find glycogen in the liver and muscles, but the level stored depends on how much training you do and your metabolism.

At any one point, there is about 4g of glucose in your blood, and the body does everything it can to maintain that – so if you fast, your muscles will release the glycogen, breaking it back down into glucose to keep your blood sugar at a steady rate. What's more, as the glycogen muscle stores break down, at the same time a process stops any more muscle glucose uptake from the blood (ensuring there is enough glucose available for all the other organs), meaning the muscles get served last.

Carbohydrates are the only macro that can be broken down quickly enough to provide you with the sustained energy you need to lift weights, which makes them pretty indispensable. They also provide the energy for muscle repair (in the form of glycogen). When you eat a meal containing carbohydrates – and this can be the starchy, slow-release carbs such as brown rice, or simple sugars which don't need to be broken down, like sweets – it is first digested in the stomach and then passes into the bloodstream. As soon as the body detects a rise in blood sugar, the brain sends a signal to the pancreas to release insulin, which makes the glucose molecules join up to make glycogen and stops any breakdown of muscle tissue. When you work out, the opposite happens: the blood glucose falls as you use the energy, and glycogen stores are broken back down (by a different hormone called glucagon) into glucose. The interesting thing about muscle glycogen is that it is not shared with any other cells and is available solely for internal use – this is why it is so important to make sure the glycogen stores are plentiful. Higher glycogen levels help you train harder for longer and allow the muscles to recover quicker. So eating carbs is a no-brainer if you want to build your muscle mass.

What you need to keep in mind is that if you consume more carbohydrates than you burn, they will be converted into triglycerides and stored as body fat for future use. That will, of course, have an impact on your body fat percentage, which will have an impact on the appearance of your physique. While excess body fat won't stop you building muscle (in fact the opposite is true – see below), it will be less visible. If the way your body or muscles look isn't part of your goals, then this isn't an issue, but if visible muscles are part of your fitness ambitions, you will need to be aware of your carb consumption as part of your overall calorie intake.

And finally, on to fat. What a chequered history fats and fitness have had. From being the absolute most evil thing you could possibly eat to now being divided up into 'clean' or 'good' fats and 'bad' fats, this macro has been the most demonised. But here's the thing: you can't live without fat in your diet. Every membrane of every cell is made of fat; fats cushion your vital organs; and 60 per cent of your brain is fat. The body cannot make its own fatty acids and without them you can't absorb vitamins and minerals, which are fat soluble. Want to know something else that's fat soluble? Hormones – including testosterone, that vital muscle-building ingredient. Without fat there is just no way you're going to build muscle anywhere near close to your potential, end of.

As our understanding of how macros work in our body progresses, we've also come to realise that fat is vital to creating that feeling of fullness. So diets that strip fat back dramatically are often doomed to fail because you will find that you're starving the entire time, and that is just not going to help you stick to your plan. And let's be honest, who wants to live like that? Conversations around good and bad fats, saturated and unsaturated fats, and good and bad cholesterol have also become so confused that many people believe it's better to just avoid fat entirely. But for most people who aren't dealing with health conditions, about 25 per cent of their overall calories should be coming from fat, and fat should be eaten with every meal, both for satiety (making you feel full) and because it lowers the gly-caemic index (i.e. how quickly each food affects your blood sugar) of the rest of what you eat. That basically means your blood sugar doesn't spike so dramatically, which is what makes you feel lethargic and hungry and can, in the long term, lead to type 2 diabetes.

The best way to calculate your daily fat intake is to multi-ply your calorie intake by 0.25, then divide by 9 (to get the amount in grams). So if you're consuming 2,500 calories a day, you'd be looking to eat 69g of fat a day (see page 119). Lisa and I get most of our fat from animal products and we also cook with coconut oil. Salmon is another good choice which we include in our diet – an average 150g fillet contains 20g of fat, while a 200g portion of chicken will provide 28g of fat.

Specifically for hypertrophy, the best way to gain strength is to be in body fat surplus. Fat is the most concentrated source of energy we have in our bodies, and people who are willing to put on body fat as well as muscle will generally get stronger quicker and gain more muscle mass because there is an abundance of energy available that the muscles can use. For people who have been raised to believe all fats lead to heart disease, it's definitely counter-intuitive that you might change your whole lifestyle and yet still gain body fat. But you have to change your perspective on the role of fat in your body. Women in particular will often ask Lisa how they can gain muscle without gaining *any* body fat, but that's basically impossible because muscle mass can only increase in a fat surplus. We often find that people, especially young women, will start gaining both muscle and the required fat to fuel that physique, and they'll decide it's not for them. The reality is that you must be prepared to put on a bit of body fat – not loads, but some.

Alternatively, you might be approaching the journey from the opposite direction, where you are carrying more body fat than you are happy with. Hopefully this will provide you with a bit of encouragement, because you are in a better position in this respect than someone who has little to no body fat when it comes to building muscle, as you are already in a fat surplus. While you won't want to increase your dietary fat consumption if you're trying to bring your body fat percentage down, you don't have to totally strip it out in the way many diets will lead you to believe – you just need to sit in a calorie deficit (see Step Three).

What might also be interesting to learn is that resistance training is now thought to have unique benefits for fat loss, as a growing number of studies suggest that weight training reshapes our metabolism. One investigation showed that people that lift weights – even occasionally – are far less likely to become obese than those that don't, while another showed that after weight training, muscles create and release little bubbles of genetic material which flow to fat cells and jump-start processes related to fat burning. What's for sure is that weightlifting in combination with a macro balanced diet and low-impact cardio (walking, for example) can reduce body fat in a sustainable, manageable way for the rest of your life. Unlike a 'fat-free' diet.

The best way to imagine the relationship between macros and muscles is like a three-legged stool: kick one leg out and you're going to massively impact the strength and balance of your platform for growth. Keep them all available as ready fuel and you're going to get the best results and make the biggest gains.

STEP THREE TO MENTAL STRENGTH: DISCIPLINE IS YOUR MOST IMPORTANT MUSCLE

***How direction, consistency and tenacity
transformed my life and body***

When it comes to improving your fitness and health, who wouldn't want to find a quick fix? The amount of work and effort that is required to alter your body composition, build muscle and reduce fat can feel completely over-whelming, especially as it often means an overhaul of your entire lifestyle. And if you want to continue to feel the benefits, those lifestyle changes are forever – they are not something you can just do for two weeks. With such a huge task ahead, it's no wonder so many people are tempted by supposed short cuts. The problem is that none of them work. Literally none of them. I see so much ter-rible advice and frankly exploitative claims on social media, trying to persuade often really vulnerable people who are struggling with their weight or body confidence to spend their money on bogus diets, supplements and fitness plans. *If it sounds too good to be true, that's because it is.* The only way to transform your body is to exercise and eat food that nourishes you and supports your body goals – and to keep doing it. There's no point pretending that it's easy. The only way you're going to be able to achieve it is through a pretty dogged sense of discipline, and that is just not easy.

Over the past decade, I've seen the power of that discipline transform my own body, health and happiness. But before I found this path I had absolutely no discipline whatsoever in any area of my life. When we see others who are fit and strong, it's easy to think they've always been that way and that you could never be like them, but from my own personal experience, that is not the case. As I mentioned in Step One, as a younger woman I didn't really know what I wanted to do as a career or what I wanted from life or my relationships. I just went with the flow, rarely speaking up or trying to guide things towards what I wanted, because I didn't know what that was. There wasn't really any need for me to have discipline – I was just bouncing along, content enough, but without any real sense of achievement or fulfilment.

93

I liked PE at school, and loved it when we did challenges like the bleep test because I do have a competitive nature when it comes to that kind of thing. I used to love sports day and doing athletics, but I was never a netball or hockey girl as I wouldn't commit to practising or getting to the matches at weekends – I just wanted to be out having fun with my friends. Discipline is such a big part of my life now, but it's something I've had to learn and make progress with, and it certainly isn't something innate. What changed for me was growing up a little bit and finding something I *really* loved. The high I got from the fitness classes was so amazing that it made me want to change my whole attitude. I got addicted to that feeling, so in a way I didn't need as much discipline to keep going back – it's obviously far harder to motivate yourself to do something you don't enjoy. I always say the first step to physical discipline is finding that niche that really gets you into exercise, because the more you like doing it, the easier it will be to keep going back. It could be yoga, martial arts or rowing – it doesn't matter as long as it's something that hooks you in. After my fitness classes, what really sealed the deal for me was weightlifting. Now weights might not be for everyone – though if you follow me on social media and have picked up this book, there's a good chance it's something you enjoy too – but don't just dismiss without trying them or because you think they aren't for women or will make you look bulky (see Step One for more discussion around this).

What I love about weightlifting is the quantifiable progress you can make. For me it's not about how big my muscles look, though obviously there is a level of gratification in actually seeing your hard work pay off – it's more about the incremental increase in my own strength. Being able to set and work towards goals in terms of what I can lift, squat, bench or press motivates me massively and helps keep me disciplined, because I know what I'm driving towards. It's like a feedback loop in that the more I improve, the more it motivates me and the less I need to rely on discipline to get me back to the weight room every day.

Obviously, there are days when I'm not feeling it, and from time to time I will fall out of my routine and lose that discipline. Like most of us, I really struggled during lockdown, and after years of consistency I totally lost my rhythm. Very quickly I lost definition in my arms, and seeing the years of hard work ebbing away felt really demoralising. That cycle can easily turn into a downward spiral if you let it, but as hard as it is to get back on track, the sooner you start, the easier it will be. And whether you're starting from square one, or trying to get back into positive habits, my approach is always the same: setting small, achievable goals is the best way to begin your journey to a healthier, happier you. Of course, you may have an overall target in the background and that's great, but focusing too much on that more often than not ends in defeat before you make it over the first hurdle. The mountain looks unconquerable from the bottom, but if you focus your gaze on the first plateau, you're more likely to set off. The steps detailed in this book aim to give you a framework to build upon, week by week. The first step might feel the hardest, but it *is* something you can achieve. From there on, it's about keeping going. Everything I recommend encompasses a lifestyle change and there are absolutely no quick fixes. I know that might not be what you want to hear, but you just can't fast-forward things. In fact, the initial foundations are so incredibly important that you won't be able to progress far without getting your form, diet and routine in place first.

In many ways, I didn't have that big a goal when I started out. I didn't really follow anyone fitness-based online, and Instagram wasn't what it is now, so I didn't have any specific ideas about what I wanted to achieve looks-wise through training and diet. These days, the women I train often say to me, 'I want to grow my glutes and quads, so I need to know which exercises to do and what I should be eating for that purpose.' Or they'll come to me with a very clear idea of what they want to get out of their training, which is really empowering and great for motivation. But at the same time, it can also be quite dispiriting if results don't come quickly or easily, and I think that having too fixed an idea in your head about how you are going to look at the 'end' can actually send you off track. I didn't really know what to expect from my classes and I kept going simply for the love of how it made my body feel rather than how it made my body look. Often the image in your head of how you will look after training is based on an image of someone else's body, and the reality is that we are all so genetically individual that you and I could do exactly the same training and eat exactly the same thing and end up looking completely different. So I would encourage you to avoid fixating on any one thing in your training, especially the way you look. More often, I suggest basing your motivation and focusing your discipline on your fitness goals. While the the way you look will inevitably be impacted by reaching your fitness goals, running that bit further, lifting that bit heavier or going that bit quicker is progress that is more objective and quantifiable.

The first few fitness classes I took were brutal. I can still remember how my body ached after doing sets and sets of squats for the first time. Because I had never moved my body like that before, I literally started from the ground, and every class felt like a huge challenge. I needed to learn all the foundations and form before I could go any further, because my body just couldn't progress without them. It's such a classic mistake to throw yourself straight into the gym, all guns blazing (probably in January with your New Year's resolutions still fresh in your mind!), but with fitness you can't just go from zero to 100, or at least not without really hurting yourself. Getting an injury is the number one thing that will hit your motivation, discipline and ultimately progress, so it is far better to focus on the smaller details. However much you want to jump forward, to get directly to where you want to be or where you used to be, you need to take it slow. Let's remember that I did five years of fitness classes before I set foot into a weight room. Now I'm not suggesting that you take it at my pace (which was more to do with confidence than anything else), but the principle of getting the fundamentals in place first – learning how to breathe, engage your muscles and not overextend your joints, for example – is vital. When that's all there, you can take the next step. And then the next and the next. By maintaining your progress that way, before you know it you will have made a huge change to your fitness – and body – without thinking about it too much or obsessing about how long it's taking you to get from A to B.

Increasing your goals over time is another way to keep feeling excited about training. Over the past decade I've shifted my targets up and up and achieved things that I would never have dreamed of. One of the biggest things I did to challenge myself was to enter a Bikini competition. Bikini Fitness is a division of competitive bodybuilding and a good starting point for anyone who is interested in competing. It was back in 2017 and Romane and I were working in LA. One day we were walking down Venice Beach, and as we were ambling down the coast, I thought about how much I needed a new challenge and how much I felt I wanted to push myself that bit further out of my comfort zone. I began to consider the idea of entering a fitness competition and wondered what it would be like. For me, the idea of stepping on to a stage and having people look at me is my worst nightmare, so while I knew the preparation would be gruelling, it was the performance element that had stopped me doing it in the past. It was definitely something the old me would *never* have done. But for some reason I just thought 'Right, now is the time to give this thing a go.'

When we got back from LA, I was ready to give it my all, which was a good thing, because it was so hard! I started off by doing a mini 'off season', which meant increasing my calories to add body fat. After ten weeks I weighed over 10 stone, which was the heaviest I'd ever been; to put it into perspective, before I started weight training I was 8 stone 3lb. This was the first time I'd ever seen myself with a bit of extra body fat on my frame. At the same time, I was training really hard. After those ten weeks, there was an eight-week cut, which meant stripping everything down and decreasing my calories while still maintaining my level of training intensity and keeping my protein intake high.

After four months, I felt like I was as ready as I was ever going to be, but I was still an absolute nervous wreck on the day of the competition. When I got up on stage my lips were trembling even when I was smiling – I had to clamp my teeth together to stop my whole face from twitching. I'd been trained in how to do all the poses, which are so much harder to master than you would think, but otherwise I did all my own make-up and got myself prepared. My tan had gone horribly wrong, and there was this lady helping to patch me up backstage, and I got into a total panic. Of course, it all worked out in the end, but my God, the adrenaline running through my body was insane. I can't remember ever having felt quite as terrified.

The competition was a qualifier for the British finals of the United Kingdom Bodybuilding and Fitness Federation (UKBFF) Championships; I came third out of seven, which meant I could progress to the finals. The feedback from the judges was that one of my quads was bigger than the other, which was a bit strange, but there's a whole culture of rules and standards that can seem overwhelming as a beginner. Even for seasoned competitors, judgements are subjective within the standards, so I didn't take it too much to heart. When I competed at the finals, I was even more nervous, because it was the biggest show in the country. And although I came last call out in the end, I was *so* happy with how I looked. Like I said, I was always just doing it for me, rather than validation from anyone else. I wasn't looking to win awards; I couldn't have cared less what any of those judges thought of me or my body. It was solely for my own sense of achievement. Looking back, I am so glad I did it, because it was such an incredible experience and it really took me forward in terms of what I believed I could accomplish. I still get a lot of confidence from knowing that I did it, even to this day, and whenever I have to do something I find challenging, like standing on a stage or speaking in front of people, I always go back to my Bikini competitions and the memories of what I managed to do there. The pictures are also epic!

If I had ever imagined that I was going to end up doing a Bikini competition back when I was a kid, I think I would have been put off any kind of fitness for life and would probably have never stepped foot in the gym in the first place. In my early twenties, I could have completely persuaded myself out of trying the weight room if I thought that kind of performance was in the future, that's how intimidated I was by it. It was far better for me to ease myself in, become confident with every little step I took and just enjoy the way the physical challenges made me feel along the way. Bit by bit, step by step I got to the point where the feeling of intimidation was outweighed by my motivation to achieve something outside of my comfort zone.

Another great side of doing Bikini was that we have clients who are prepping for all sorts of competitions and the experience meant that I can now really empathise and understand what they are going through, which ultimately has made me better at doing my job. I'm able to give them so much more support than I would otherwise have been able to. It would have been easy to think, 'Oh, I'm qualified as a PT now, and anything I don't know I can just ask Romane.' But that is not how my brain is programmed. Having discipline in my life has meant that I never want to rest on my laurels and just coast along being OK at something. I spent years of my life not pushing myself, never knowing what I could achieve, and as much as I don't regret the fun I had with my friends and family during that time, it's incomparable to the fulfilment I now have in my life. It's almost as if the discipline I've gained from my physical practice has rewired my brain, and that has a huge impact on the way I live my life. I'm never not going to want to be better at what I do.

Fitness has definitely helped me to believe in myself and push myself to do things that I would never have done before. That's the amazing thing about the relationship between physical and mental strength – by building one, you inevitably build the other, often without even really thinking about it. Just as my body has developed over time, so my mental strength has become more and more resilient. When I think back to my school days and how discipline was presented as something really boring, I had no idea it could be such a force for change. Now I would say that I'm actually a routine kind of person. Creating a clear routine and rhythm to my days and weeks has really helped me with my discipline and makes getting to the gym and sticking to my nutritional goals much more manageable. Of course, sometimes I do eat something which isn't 'optimum' for strength training – I'm not a monk, and I absolutely believe that if you deny yourself everything, it's not sustainable.

What you tell yourself in your head has a huge impact on your ability to be consistent and take the steps you want and need to reach your goals. If I think, 'I can't be bothered to go to the gym, I'm not really feeling it today,' it's incredibly hard to pull back from that. And the next day it's really easy to say the same thing. And the next, and so on. But if

I wake up and feel off, but say to myself, 'I feel rubbish, but the gym is going to make me feel so much better,' it's easier to motivate myself to get there. Who doesn't want to feel better? Of course, there are days when you do need a break – if you've got a bit of gym fatigue, obviously it's good to take a bit of time out. But speaking from recent experience, a day here or there is fine, but when the days start to roll into weeks, it can be really tough to stop the spiral gathering pace. Getting back into the gym after lockdown felt like I was almost back to square one, and made me remember what it was like to be a beginner again.

The way I deal with that situation is to ease myself back in and not try to hit it on day one. Mentally, I prepare to re-establish my rhythm by honing the short-term goals and giving myself a realistic time frame for achieving them. There is nothing like ticking off boxes – whether they're in your mind or written down in a journal. If you go back into the gym after a lapse in discipline and think you're going to magically get back to where you were, you're going to be massively disappointed (and sore, too). It's like looking at the mountain and focusing on the big picture again. You *will* get back to where you were, you will even go beyond where you were, but to begin with you have to step back and reset your foundations. Time flies when you're on the path to achieving what you really want, and before you

know it you'll be looking down from the top of that mountain again.

I mentioned earlier how important it is to invest in your
physical strength for the right reasons, and I really believe
that you won't get the same kind of mental strength pay-off
if you are working out for someone else. Though I started
going to the gym because of something someone said to
me, and then let my partner's opinion affect the type of
exercise I did, over time I have been able to shed any outside influences on my personal physical development. The
mental cues that get women to the gym include thinking
that a partner will like you more if you are thinner/ have a
smaller waist/ bigger bum and thighs, and so on. You might
feel that you will be more likely to find a partner if you
change the way you look. Perhaps someone in your family
has said something about your body and it's made you feel
you need to change yourself to win their acceptance. Or
maybe it was a 'friend' or colleague. Maybe you feel pressure to lose weight after having a baby or another life event.
Of course, you may still be able to motivate yourself to
work out and change your diet and lifestyle for these reasons, but over time it is very hard to keep up your discipline
if all the effort is for someone else. Trying to alter your body
to suit someone else's standards and perceptions presents so
many issues. What if your body isn't built to look the way

they want it to? What if you gain muscle in areas that they don't like? What if you make the changes and it's still not enough for them to love you or accept you? When it comes down to it, anyone who asks you to change for any reason other than improving your health will probably never be satisfied.

Changing your physical self for someone else also means you are starting from a really negative place mentally, and when results are slow to come (which they can be for all of us), you can quickly become disenchanted, which often leads to a fall-off in discipline. How can you expect to grow your own self-esteem and confidence when you are doing everything to please someone else? To gain mental strength, the only person you need to prove anything to is yourself. That's why I believe it is so important to start your fitness journey from a place of self-motivation. If it is purely a challenge for yourself and against yourself, you will reap the full physical and mental rewards. How far you can push yourself, which goals you hit and how strong you can become are things you will have to dig deep inside to find out. If you don't really want to do it, or you only want to do it to make someone else happy, you're not going to get the same results.

This is why I also encourage you to try to forget about your looks when you are building your strength. Obviously, a lot of people go to the gym because they don't like the way they look, and as a woman who has always been slim and enjoyed the privileges that come with that, I'm in no position to criticise that. But if you don't enjoy the process, you are much less likely to get to the finish line. I absolutely am not saying that there is anything wrong with going to the gym to lose body fat, for example. If that is what will improve your confidence and lead you on the path to a healthier lifestyle, that is wonderful. However, just focusing on the numbers on the scales or the dress size you fit into won't sustain the lifelong lifestyle change that you need to maintain a strong body and mind. I have also never seen the point in letting a number determine how you feel. Enjoying the elation that exercise gives you (that addictive endorphin high), embracing your new strength and finding confidence in your new abilities will make the actual process of getting up, making it to the mat and actually doing the exercise so much more enjoyable. The truth is, the less discipline you need to keep your routine going, the easier it will be to be consistent, which is the most important aspect of any training plan.

Since entering the weight room for the first time, I have only fallen more in love with fitness. Not for anyone else, but for myself. It's where I built myself back up from being made to feel worthless, and where I found my confidence and self-love. It's where I feel my strongest and it has become my safe place, where my time is for *me* and no one can take that away (what a freaking feeling!). All of that has nothing to do with the way I look and everything to do with how I feel about having achieved my goals through commitment and hard work. And that is what I want for you too.

Building a strong community around you is one thing you can do to help support your discipline. While I do believe that ultimately change comes from within, that doesn't mean you have to do it all on your own, or that you can't lean on others along the way. That is one of the reasons I decided to set up my app, and I am so proud of the incredible communities who have connected with each other on Facebook especially, but also on Instagram and TikTok. My number one ambition when I decided that I was going to give my all to a career in fitness was to create something that could help people. Seeing the community around @LisaFitt and Strong & Sxy has been the most rewarding aspect of my years in the industry, and that is what I want to develop even further as I know it means so much to so many people. Having a community that you can talk to, ask for advice and share your vulnerabilities and challenges with can make all the difference when it comes to maintaining your discipline. The encouragement of other people in my life, especially Romane, has kept me focused on my goals and helped me achieve things that I could never otherwise have dreamed of. You only have to look at the threads and conversations in my communities to see the value of having like-minded people on the same journey around you. Lifting each other up through the hard times, inspiring each other to go further, sharing motivation and tips for everything from workouts to recipes and mental health, a strong community can act like a backbone for your discipline and scoop you up when your strength wavers. None of us are machines, and sometimes you just need that human touch and reassurance to keep you going.

As for my own motivation and goals, there is still so much for me to do. It's been twelve years now since I took that first exercise class, and I'm still so passionate about fitness and what I'm doing. There's that saying that turning your hobby into a job will ruin it for you, but that is so far from the case with me. I still love lifting weights every single day, and Romane and I are still just as enthusiastic about what we're building. It can certainly be exhausting, putting your heart and soul into a business, and taking big leaps of faith is really tough because I second-guess things all the time, but I am getting better and better at believing in myself and feeling confident in the future.

One of the biggest risks we have taken to date was launching our app. Romane first started talking about the idea back in 2018, before we had seen anyone else do a successful fitness app. I remember saying absolutely no way to the idea and thinking he was crazy. At that point I didn't have the following that I do now and I just didn't have the understanding of the value of the app to both our business and to my followers. I also didn't think anyone would download it – low-balling myself, as usual. But once I'd started doing my workout videos and it was clear how useful they were and how much everyone loved them, the idea came up again, and this time I felt ready to take the plunge. I am still inherently cautious and that will always be part of my make-up. But the more I achieve, the more comfortable I am with the discomfort of risk-taking. It costs a shitload of money to build an app, along with so much hard work and time. I wanted it to be absolutely seamless, and definitely didn't want it to be one of those apps you downloaded and never thought about again. So we spent the whole of 2019 designing, creating and testing it, and sometimes I found it a challenge to stay focused. I ended up using a lot of the lessons learned from my time in the gym to help me. Instead of constantly worrying about the whole app and how on earth we would ever get it finished, I chopped it all down into more manageable bite-sized tasks and set about ticking them off my list. At times it felt like I was drowning, as I was trying to manage my other workload too, but it ended up being worth every single late night and stressful deadline.

By consolidating everything that we had worked for into one place, it took our business up to the next level. And we got really lucky with timing. Launching in January 2020, we had absolutely no idea that the world was about to be plunged into lockdown and that everyone would be desperate for at-home workouts (in fact we almost didn't include an at-home section!). By early March, the app was being used 90 per cent in gyms and only 10 per cent at home, but as soon as we went into lockdown, it just flipped the other way. The fact that the at-home content had been an afterthought seems crazy in retrospect, but who could have predicted what was coming? Aside from well-considered home workouts and tips for maximising the effectiveness of training without gym fitness equipment, the app also offers nutritional advice with bespoke plans created by our own STRNG-certified nutritionist – all of which was really useful during the pandemic as so many people struggled with keeping healthy over the year.

What the experience with the app taught me once again was that when you believe in yourself and stay committed to seeing something through, amazing things can happen.

We could so easily have put off building the app as I had so much else on my plate. It was also such a slog putting it all together that we could have been completely derailed if we hadn't stayed disciplined. If I had focused too much on the mountain instead of the manageable short-term goals, I would probably have been overwhelmed. But to have missed the moment would have been heartbreaking for our business, and would also have meant that the thousands of people we helped to stay fit and healthy during such an intense and unsettling time wouldn't have had our guidance or the support of the amazing community that has built up around the app.

The discipline I have built in the weight room led to me achieving my body goals. That achievement led in turn to an increase in confidence. That increased confidence made me believe in myself more and more over time, and that gave me the guts to take a massive business risk. My discipline stepped back in and kept me on track to complete the work needed to launch the app, while the lessons I'd learned in the gym of tackling a mammoth task step by step gave me a framework with which to manage the huge workload I had to get through. When I talk about how your steps to physical strength go hand in hand with mental strength, and how they both contribute to a positive and successful future, that is exactly what I mean.

I look back and think of myself in my twenties and how lost I was. If I hadn't started my fitness classes, then got into weightlifting, the following things are certain:

1. I wouldn't have set up an Instagram account
2. I wouldn't have met the love of my life
3. I wouldn't have started my own business
4. I wouldn't be travelling around the world for my work
5. I wouldn't have gained self-confidence and learned to love myself
6. I wouldn't be anywhere near as happy
7. I wouldn't have fulfilled a fraction of my potential

It's very easy to dismiss going to the gym as just a leisure activity. Of course, you can take a lot of pleasure from it and it can be a massive de-stressor in the middle of a busy week. But maintaining a fit and healthy body is about so much more than just taking a break from work or kids. For me, it has been the key to unlocking a completely different and so much happier life.

I'm not saying that weightlifting is going to 100 per cent lead to the exact seven points above for you. But there is no doubt in my mind that the physical and mental strength that come with it will change the trajectory of your life for the better. So what are you waiting for?!

STEP THREE RECAP:

- Forget about the quick fix. When it comes to health and fitness, physical and mental strength, there are no short cuts, you just have to do the work. Be wary of anyone selling you a magic recipe for progress without effort, and remember that there are countless people out there willing to exploit others. The fitness world on social media is a bit like the Wild West, so always do your research, read testimonials and follow a creator for some time before trusting anyone.

- Discipline isn't something you either have or don't. It's something you have to invest in and build over time. It has the power to totally transform your body, mind and life, but it is by no means straightforward. You have to keep working at it – just like everyone else, I've gone through times when my discipline has gone to crap.

- Physical discipline will lead to mental discipline and vice versa. It's an endless feedback loop, supporting and stretching your potential every single day.

- There's only one person you need to prove yourself to: you. Training for yourself will boost your mental strength and that in turn will be transformative for your entire life.

- Keep pushing yourself outside of your comfort zone. Discipline helps you progress towards your goals, which should be ever-shifting. There is no 'end' to your diet or fitness routine; instead it's a new lifestyle which will lead you to do things that you never believed yourself capable of (like the Bikini competition for me!).

STEP THREE TO PHYSICAL STRENGTH: THE CALORIE QUESTION

To count or not to count?

Romane

We've become so used to hearing about calories that it's difficult to remember what they actually are. Calories, or kcals, have been the subject of endless articles, books and Instagram lives, and there seems to be no aspect of the calorie debate that hasn't stoked some kind of controversy. People will tell you that it doesn't matter what you eat as long as you count your calories; that a calorie is a calorie; that calories don't matter anyway, it's all about your balance of macros (which usually involves excluding one or the other). Others will insist that calories are old-fashioned, and that everything depends on your gut microbiome (the bacteria

118

in your intestines) or your genetic make-up. And one of the biggest problems is that there is evidence to support pretty much all of the above.

So, let's dial back. What do we mean by a kcal? One calorie is the amount of energy needed to raise the temperature of 1kg of water by 1 degree. That's where the k comes from and, yes, it's literally that simple. Fats have 9 kcals per gram, whereas carbohydrates and proteins have 4 kcals per gram. The number of calories we burn per day varies dramatically due to a broad range of elements – some genetic, some environmental – and hard as it is to accept, that means that part of it is out of your control. What is true for all of us, though, is that without consuming calories as fuel, we wouldn't be able to do anything. Just to keep our heart beating, our lungs breathing, and our brain functioning, calories are our petrol and our bodies are thirsty engines.

The basic story has always been that if you want to lose body fat, you need to be in a calorie deficit, whereas if you want to gain body fat, you need to be in a calorie surplus. The tricky element is calculating your individual daily maintenance calories. Starting with your BMR (Basal Metabolic Rate) – the number of calories you need simply to survive – you then add on the kcals you burn through activity to reach your overall calorie expenditure. How you calculate your BMR is contested, but there are several equations out there: the Harris Benedict, Katch McArdle and the Mifflin St Jeor. (I'm not taking the piss here, these are actually the names of formulae!) I use a Fitbit, which isn't perfect, but gives you an idea to within 15 per cent and I find it really useful.

Once you've worked out your approximate personal expenditure, you're in a position to start building your own nutrition plan. What is clear to us, through our work with clients over the years, is that when it comes to building muscle mass, most people don't realise they need to eat for the body they want, not the body they have. And because generations of health messaging has emphasised fat loss and highly restrictive diets, most people undereat when they start training, sometimes dramatically.

If Lisa wanted to build more muscle, she would have to eat a calorie surplus beyond her daily 2,500 for a long while to get past where she is now. For me, I burn around 5,000 calories a day, which is obviously way more than you'll ever be told to eat in any conventional diet. The reality is that our active lifestyle – for me three or four hours running around the gym filming Lisa, hours of training, then cardio – means we burn an incredible number of calories. Someone who has an active job, such as on a building site, might tell us they eat loads but just can't put any muscle mass on. Well, sure, they might eat a big breakfast in the caff in the morning and a big dinner, but only a sandwich and crisps for lunch, so maybe they eat 2,500 calories overall. It's just not enough to fuel muscle creation.

What the government daily calorie advice doesn't take into account are activity levels, especially when it comes to weightlifting. The biggest response we got when we initially launched our app was from people sceptical and worried about the amount of food we were recommending they ate. We had endless messages, from women in particular, asking how they could possibly eat that much, saying that we were recommending too many calories and that there must be something wrong with the app. It didn't come as a surprise, because most diets tell you to eat 1,000–1,500 calories per day to get into shape, and that's generally what people are used to reading. What they don't realise is that to build muscle you need that surplus, and you absolutely need to make sure there are ready nutrients in your body to fuel hypertrophy.

I can't say it loudly enough: if you want to build muscle, you have to eat food! If you want to look like Lisa, make gains, have energy for the gym and to make the lifts, you have to eat. Women who actually lift and are strong with a good amount of muscle mass – they all eat. You have to fully nourish your body rather than restrict your food. That is why Lisa looks so healthy – her skin glows because she is nourished (and hydrated) with everything her body needs.

The margins that you find in regular diets, where you're encouraged to shave 500, even 1,000 calories off your daily expenditure, are not the same when you lift. When you're regularly doing resistance training, if you want to drop body fat, you need to be in deficit by about 300 calories a day. Conversely, if you want to gain muscle, you need to be in a calorie surplus of about 300 calories a day. As you can see, the margins are very small and that is why we continue to weigh our food.

Here we need to take a little pause to address the elephant in the room: counting calories is not appropriate for everyone, especially if you have had control issues or experiences with disordered eating. I would never ever suggest that anyone weigh their food down to the last gram, or lie awake at night totting up the calories they have eaten each day. But for some people, even a more casual approach to recording food intake can lead to behaviours that are detrimental to your happiness and health. And let's always remember, that's what this is about. If you have struggled in any way with these issues, I always recommend you work with a specialist to create a nutritional set-up that takes into account your specific needs and helps you work through any lingering mental health concerns.

If you feel comfortable with this, it is definitely worth investing in a food scale. If you have a physical goal, whether that is body fat loss or muscle gain, weighing your food is extremely useful. If you've been running endlessly on the treadmill, or lifting more and more weight and seeing no progress, it could be because you have been giving yourself larger or smaller portions than you thought. Even now, after so many years, I still can't totally guesstimate. While it's completely understandable that food weighing has had a bad press, for those who have never had any food issues, it's definitely worth considering.

To try and keep a sense of balance and not feel under too much pressure, I recommend looking at the week as a whole when it comes to calculating calories, rather than obsessing over every single day. For five days a week, Lisa and I will be in deficit, but we top that up on Wednesdays and Saturdays, when Lisa might consume 3–4,000 calories to push her into overall surplus to fuel progression for the week. At the moment, I generally do all the cooking, because I just love giving people that feeling of a good meal and making them feel happy and it's one of the best ways I know to support Lisa, but we've gone through periods where she has done the cooking – it's just swings and roundabouts for us really, being there for each other whenever we can. Every morning when I wake up, I weigh and prep the food for both of us for the day. It's not like I'm serving up crazy, fancy meals six times a day – we eat the same effective, simple meals every day, like Cajun chicken and rice, which has become a real staple for us. It suits our lifestyle to stick to things which are consistent but tasty. That might sound quite boring, but we love it and find it so beneficial for our results. Obviously, we know that not everyone is like us, and our app is full of adventurous recipe ideas, but I do think there is value in keeping things simple in general.

As for the balance of calories per macro, you want to be eating at least 1g of protein per pound of weight, around 25 per cent of your calories should come from fat, and the rest of your target calories from carbohydrates. In this balance, a 130lb woman (Lisa's weight), training consistently through the week, should be eating around 2,500 kcals per day: 150g of protein, 70g of fat and the remaining calories from carbohydrate sources.

The jury is still out on whether it makes any difference if the food is processed or not, but we try and stick to unprocessed foods and will always choose whole foods where we can. For us, preparation is key. If we don't have our meals ready, we will generally have a really shit day, not only because are we hangry, scurrying around thinking about what we can eat, but because we then have no energy when we get to the gym, which will really annoy us both. If we are away, or if we go out for the day, we always bring our food with us. That doesn't mean that we might not decide to have lunch in a restaurant, but we will never be caught short. We like to be prepared and we don't like to be hungry. Ever! For some people this might seem too strict, but it's what keeps us consistent and on track with our goals.

If we do go to a restaurant, we are mindful that there should be protein, carbs and fats on the plate, but in general we have whatever we fancy. If we have a bit of extra fat one day, we'll just get up earlier the next day and do some walking, or do a bit more exercise when we get to the gym. I guess what I want to get across is that it isn't stressful – we don't feel anxious about our food and our training, and it doesn't ever feel like a chore; we just enjoy it all. When you change your lifestyle and start on a path towards a final goal, a lot of this becomes second nature. All you need is preparation and consistency, with a diet that feeds your training and fuels your muscles to grow.

On days when you feel you have overpitched your calorie target, don't panic. One of the worst things you can do for your muscle gain is to believe you need to hit the gym super-hard and beast yourself with back-to-back HIIT classes. While there is a place for cardio, over a relatively short space of time it will start to undermine your muscle mass. The sweet spot is finding the fat-burning zone with low-intensity, steady cardio options like walking. As Lisa has a natural ectomorph body type, she has to be particularly aware of this, as a lot of high-intensity exercise would very quickly start to eat into her muscle gain. When she was doing the live workouts during lockdown, she found it much harder to maintain her muscle mass, so do try to resist the urge to try and work off any extra calories in a frenzied gym session.

The goal with your diet overall is the same as your goal in the gym: a new lifestyle which supports you to achieve a stronger body and mind for good. This isn't a six-week programme, it's a for-the-rest-of-your-life programme. A day here or there means nothing when you have a great structure in place, so leave the sweating for the gym!

STEP FOUR TO MENTAL STRENGTH: KNOW WHEN TO TAKE YOURSELF SERIOUSLY

And when to really not ... !

Of the many run-ins I had with bosses in my previous work life, one stands out for being particularly nasty. I was working at a small company and I had become really tight with one other employee (probably because we thought the boss was such a tyrant). We were constantly joking and taking the mick out of each other, but one day he told me that our boss had said something really out of order about me: 'The thing with Lisa is that you can tell she will never make more than £16,000.' Now, I'm not money-minded, so it wasn't the actual numbers that stung, it was more the idea that people around me felt I would never amount to anything, that I had no future or potential to ever be a success. Because I'd done badly in my GCSEs and came from a modest background, it was like he'd written me off at twenty years old. Truth be told, I believed the same: I didn't think I would ever earn a good salary or deserve to be promoted or be successful in my career. His words just confirmed what I already thought about myself – I was nothing, and no one would ever take me seriously at work; I was always going to be on the bottom rung of the ladder. Having a complete lack of self-esteem and feeling so small in nearly all environments meant that I didn't back myself at all. So much so that I couldn't even identify with my inner voice, couldn't even acknowledge that I had an ambition or hopes or dreams for myself. I was just Lisa from Dunstable and, outside of my friends and family, I felt I would never matter.

When you walk around feeling that way about yourself, that is what you project. If you don't believe in yourself – that you are worthy of love or investment or anyone else's support – why would anyone else believe in you? It's basically a self-fulfilling prophecy: when you don't believe your voice counts, no one bothers to listen when you talk. Developing self-belief has been the mental struggle of my life. It remains a constant work in progress, and I have crises of confidence and lose my footing fairly often. But sometimes I catch myself talking down to myself and manage to stop myself in my tracks. What I've built in the gym, what I've built in my business and what I've built in my marriage are all things to be proud of, and they have all helped to take me from ground zero in terms of confidence to a place where I hold my own.

So where do you start if you want to turn the tide in your own battle for self-belief? If I could go back in time and speak to my eighteen-year-old self, the first thing I would say is to find something that you believe in. It could be literally anything, but a life without any kind of passion is always going to be unfulfilled. I would then say, forget everything you've been told about education. I got terrible GCSE results, and so did Romane, but that hasn't stopped us from building and running a really successful business. Being academic and being successful are two very different things. You don't need a degree to set up a business (just ask Bill Gates, Richard Branson, Oprah ...), and the one-size-fits-all approach of schools is just rubbish. It's never too late to start something new or create something you believe in – whether that's after a first career or after having children. This idea that by twenty-five we should all be on the path to incredible success, and if we're not it means we're doomed to a mediocre career (and life), is so damaging. I know that many people feel exactly the same: that somehow because of their background, academic limitations or general lack of obvious skills, they will never achieve anything significant.

But you can't let these kinds of flawed ideas hold you back. There is no one in the world 'like you' and, what's more, people from your background with your school grades have gone on to achieve amazing things, and you can too.

The one thing you do need to get you from A to B, however, is a shitload of hard work. There is absolutely no point pretending that anything I have achieved has been easy, or that the self-belief I've built off the back of those achievements was gained in a straightforward way. But when you find your passion and work incredibly hard at it, you can build professional success. Obviously, there will be hurdles to jump (I'm still jumping them every week!), and you have to prepare yourself for setbacks and hard times. But just because you don't have five A-grades, it doesn't mean you should waste your life doing something that's unfulfilling because you think that's all you're good for. You can always learn, develop and become better at something you are passionate about – that's just the law of returns. For years I trod water, believing I wasn't worth anything more. I completely internalised what my school, my ex-boyfriends and my bosses told me about myself and couldn't imagine another path. But I still managed to turn it around and end up where I am today – which is way beyond my craziest expectations. Currently our business employs and supports eight people in addition to me and

131

Romane. I have millions of people following my business and progress on Instagram, 18,000 active members of our Facebook group, and tens of thousands of men and women training with my videos and through our app. We'll soon be launching our very own supplement service, I'm writing my own goddam book ... and who knows what will be next? It's absolutely wild.

Perhaps wilder still is the fact that even with all this validation and tangible proof of my worth, I continue to struggle with it. Even to this day, I'm still not the one that takes charge in meetings or takes the lead with our business, and I definitely don't see myself as this big, shiny entrepreneur. I'm never going to be rushing to do a PowerPoint presentation or get up on stage to speak to an audience; there are still a bunch of things that feel impossible for me. But now, due to the confidence I've gained over the years, I won't stay silent if I have a point to make, and that is such huge progress for me. While I would still never put myself in any position that would feel confrontational, I have definitely found the courage to speak up for myself, especially when I have a really clear gut instinct about something. I've learned over the years not to bottle things up for too long. That's something that runs in my family, especially in my dad, but the problem with not saying or doing something when you really feel it deep in your gut is that you're setting yourself up for regret further down the line. The number of times I've thought 'Damn, I knew this would happen, I should have said something ... ' – but now, as soon as I get that pang in my gut, I *will* say something. It still takes a lot for me to feel comfortable enough to speak freely and with conviction, and it often means it takes a lot of time until I trust people. But I'm getting there.

One of the biggest problems I've always had in terms of getting myself heard is with the actual volume of my voice. When I go to restaurants, or order at a counter, nine times out of ten I'll be asked to repeat what I've said, something which makes me feel incredibly shy and embarrassed. I'll then be even quieter, usually until one of my friends or Romane ends up ordering for me! I'm the same on Zoom – often I speak so quietly that the microphone doesn't pick up my voice and the person on the other end has to ask me to repeat myself. I don't know if I will ever grow out of it, because it's something I've done my whole life. It does knock my confidence and make me wonder what's wrong with me and why I speak so softly, but it's obviously something to do with my struggles with self-belief. As I've said before, I'm still a work in progress, but the important thing to note is that even with issues such as these, you can still be a success if you play to your strengths and have a great team behind you.

I definitely still bear the scars of my past, but some of my anxiety comes from more recent experiences, and some of it from my new career in social media. When I say more recent experiences, what I really mean is that even now people sometimes take a dislike to me, though they know nothing about me, and that continues to turn me inside out. I want to be able to say that I don't care what other people think about me, but the problem is that when you're constantly fighting off negative thoughts about yourself from within, when someone else criticises you, all it does is serve to reconfirm the negativity.

Romane and I recently started attending a new gym, and I got chatting to someone who had initially been really friendly. We'd shared skincare tips and I thought we had been getting on really well. Then, from nowhere, they started completely blanking me and wouldn't even acknowledge me, which was pretty awkward considering we were in the gym every day. They blocked me on social media and had obviously completely taken against me. I know, logically speaking, that I hadn't done anything to justify that kind of treatment – but it follows a pattern that has been repeated throughout my life.

Since I started working on social media, these kinds of issues have taken on a deeper significance, because I now wonder if someone has taken against me because I work as

134

an 'influencer', and if they dislike me because of something they have seen on my account. Before that, no one knew who I was, so issues could only stem from knowing me in person. This extra layer has transformed my worries about meeting new people into a real anxiety. I find myself think-ing, maybe they don't like me because of what I do for a living. Maybe they think I'm fake or that my content is shit. Maybe I posted something that annoyed them.

Plenty of people don't take a career built through social media seriously. They think our lives are easy, and that all we do is ponce around the gym taking selfies all day long. When Romane and I first started our business there were even friends and close family members who weren't always supportive of what we were doing. It's understandable that some people don't get it – it is definitely new and unfamiliar territory. But often people didn't even try or want to under-stand – it was as though, because we weren't following the 'rules' of how things should be done, they couldn't see the work we were putting in. Going to the gym for us is *work*. End of! That is how we promote our services, it's where we make content, it's where I build my following. Some people thought we were just dossers, because for them going to the gym was a leisure activity, something you did on your day off. We were also judged for moving back to my mum and dad's to save some money. I suppose from the outside it might have looked like we were sponging off my family – we were in our late twenties, spending all day in the gym while not paying rent, so I guess they came to the conclusion that we must be work-shy drifters. Obviously, my mum and dad saw all the hard work we were putting in, and we were so grateful that they wanted to support our plans for the future. But it still got to me that so many people around us thought we were a bit of a joke.

Not only were Romane and I working all hours to get the business off the ground, but he was also competing a lot at the time and we were really burning the candle at both ends. Nearly all of our friends and family were working 9–5 Monday–Friday, so they just had no idea of the amount of graft that was going on behind the scenes.

There was this sense that we were wasting our time and should just get 'proper' jobs. I really don't think it was meant in a horrible way – those close to us were just concerned that things wouldn't work out and they didn't want to see us land on our asses. It took Romane's mum a long time to get her head around our career. She just couldn't believe that we were working hard, because for her, success and hard work went hand in hand with a stable, salaried job. It wasn't until recently that she really saw how much had gone into what we've built from nothing. When we bought our house and she came to stay for the first time, I think the penny dropped. She could finally see the hours that we dedicated to our job, and I think that helped her understand that it was a legitimate business. Obviously, now people have been able to see the end results, their attitudes have changed. Our friends and families are really proud of us, and have made an effort to try and understand how this new world works. But it was a long time coming. Sometimes you can't wait for other people to take you seriously and even the people that love you the most won't always have the imagination to be able to see where you are going. It's really horrible to have people think that you are a bum when you are putting everything you have into your work, but when you start something new, there will always be people who either try to put you down because it threatens their idea of how things should be done, or else tell you to go back to the old way because they worry the risk is too great. Staying strong in the face of that and focusing on our daily goals was the only way we could rise above it.

Another issue we faced was the belief that if you're working on social media, you're a total fraud, just out to make a quick buck. As a genuine person who is very loyal and transparent, I do find it tricky to be part of an industry where there is a lot of inauthenticity and exploitation. Because outrageous things do happen in the influencer world, people don't believe that you could have morals and act in good faith. I know that I'm a good person, but it can be so difficult when people accuse you of things you patently haven't done. It is hard to be tarred with the same brush as those who really are in it only for what they can get, and it's tough that the word 'influencer' has got such a bad rap. Ultimately, there isn't a different way to describe what I do – I post content on social media, and my social platforms drive sales of my meal and training plans, app and other products. But the amount of hard work and commitment that has gone into every tiny thing I've put my name to is insane, and as far away as possible from blagging. I would really hope that it is obvious that what I do is different to, say, someone coming straight off a reality show and just advertising anything they can for 'easy money'. I do think that Romane and I have done a very good job over the years of being entirely transparent. I have always been truthful, and I've never had anything to hide from my followers, so I know there's nothing any-one can dig up about me and put out there. But it does feel like you have to constantly justify yourself and prove that what you are doing has good intentions, and that can take its toll.

Last year there was a particularly difficult moment, which made me reconsider a lot of the ways in which I was work-ing. I had been selling my resistance bands through the app and they had been a bit of slow burner. Then Covid-19 hit, and everyone was desperate to buy cheap equipment for at-home exercise. Almost overnight we sold out, and as they took weeks to restock, we couldn't fulfil the demand. Because people were so desperate, we decided that we would offer a pre-order, so that as soon as the new bands arrived, they would be dispatched to people who really wanted them. What we hadn't factored in was how the worldwide shipping issues on top of Covid would impact the delivery. We had assumed that by doubling the usual delivery time we would be well covered, but when it came to it, some people didn't receive their bands in the promised time. Now, don't get me wrong, customers totally deserve to express their disappointment – I would feel the same. But the level of vitriol was just explosive.

Social media can be a volatile place anyway, because of the anonymity and general heated tone at times. But I really hadn't expected it to blow up in the way it did. I understand that as the face of my business, people are going to come to me and express their feelings, both positive and negative – that is just the nature of things. But by the end of that week, my inbox was rammed with aggressive messages accusing me of being a money-grabbing con artist, and that's putting it politely. Every post I put up would be met with comments saying such negative things about me and the business. I've always done what I do for the passion and enjoyment that I get through helping others. If the money comes in, that's wonderful, but I was fine earning an average salary and I would be fine on that again. So to see people all over my account so unhappy with my service and so disappointed in me personally, based on the idea that I had cheated them out of money, was crushing.

From a mental health perspective everything snowballed for me. The problem was that I was waking up first thing in the morning and barely finishing my coffee before reading my DMs and being overwhelmed with the attacks and criticism. I'm such a routine person, so every day I was starting things off exactly the same by replying to endless messages, which were generally all negative (understand-able) and sometimes hate-filled (less so). Of course there were those who were perfectly civil and understanding. But others used the opportunity to offload in a way they wouldn't have if they were speaking to you in real life. For the whole day my mood would be really, really down. At first I couldn't work out why I was feeling so low day in and day out; then I realised I was starting every morning feel-ing so miserable about something I had no control over. Trying to get back to all the people reaching out had been like fighting a losing battle for a long time – 2.5 million followers equates to a lot of messages – and with the bands debacle on top of that, I finally made the decision that I needed to share the workload of managing my account. I just couldn't do it on my own anymore.

When I'm down, it's hard to find the motivation to push myself and the business forward, to make great content, to come up with new ideas and bring the good energy that I need for everything that I'm doing. During this time, I lost all my drive and positivity, and when you're not just financially supporting yourself, but also looking after the wages and mortgages of other people and their families, your investment in your own mental health goes beyond self-care. I didn't have a choice but to take my mental health seriously, or else my entire business and everyone who worked there would have suffered too. Knowing that you have people relying on you can be a really big weight, and it's not something I take lightly in any way, so I needed to find a solution. Now I have a team member who looks after all my platforms and deletes abusive messages. It takes a fair amount of time every day to remove the obscene and offensive content that is sent, and knowing that's the case does feel like a kick to the stomach. But having a barrier between myself and those words definitely helps. The truth is that people can say anything on social media and you can't predict how it's going to make you feel. Some days I might be able to brush something off and not even think about it again, but sometimes it will get to me and eat me up all day, undermining my ability to be anywhere near my best self. I still have a sensitive soul and my job makes it particularly difficult because the online world is full of people with opinions.

My hope is that I can get to a place of acceptance and fully take on board that when people treat me badly without knowing me, either on- or offline, it's their problem not mine. When I really think about it and remove my instinctive habit of believing all criticism levelled against me, I do know that it can't be down to anything I've done and that it's not my fault. I think so many of us have this unquenchable desire to be liked, and because of that find social media a really tricky space. I'm a bloody people pleaser, and always want to make others feel happy, so it can be hard to take when people are so vocal in their dislike of you. However, I have learned that when someone is negative towards me on social media in particular, it's often because they're sad in their own lives, which isn't a nice thing to think about. Now, if I do come across a negative comment myself, I'll always reply nicely and wish them well, because I actually end up feeling sorry for their situation. If you need to bring someone else down to make yourself feel better, it's not a great place to be.

There are, of course, times when I see other people who work in my industry at events and exhibitions, and I have definitely wound myself up about that in the past and felt my heart race at the thought of having to speak to so many new people in such a big crowd. Some people go to these events with a clear agenda of who they are going to speak to based on their following, or try to make collaborations happen with people they believe can further their business. There is definitely a lot of faux friendliness, but I think I've developed a strong radar for it now, and because I'm naturally guarded I've never really had an issue with anyone in my industry and nothing bad has ever happened to me at an event. I prefer to just go with the flow and thus far, I've always found everyone to be super-welcoming. In the back of my mind there is a small, cynical voice that wonders if people are only so kind because I have a lot of followers. There is also a strange disconnect, in the sense of not knowing what people are going to be like in real life in comparison to how they are online. I have met people who are quite clearly acting the entire time on social media, because in real life they are completely different. I also have moments of self-awareness, when I wonder how the hell it's possible that I am here with all these amazing athletes and inspirational men and women who I look up to. I have to shake myself and remind myself that I have worked hard to be here too.

It's a funny one, because I never set out to be where I am today. I never thought, 'I'm going to be CEO of a business which employs a team of people.' Or, 'I'm going to build a business with customers across the world.' Nothing was premeditated and I never set myself unrealistic goals – what has happened is the result of me loving what I do. I don't think I had an ounce of entrepreneurial spirit at the beginning. I remember when the medium told me I was going to have my own business in the fitness industry, and it was just laughable as I really believed it wasn't in my blood. The thing that has made it manageable is the way we have built the business step by tiny step – the same way that I built my body. And after each progression, it's felt more and more do-able to push that bit further. It would be impossible to have gone through all of this and not have gained at least a bit of self-esteem, because it takes so much out of you to keep going. And because of that I am starting to take myself and my achievements a little more seriously, because I am so proud of what Romane and I have built over the past six years. I'm starting to feel vindicated for all the decisions we've made and proud of everyone we've proved wrong. (Who's calling who a dosser now?!)

But I will never stray too far from self-deprecation. I mean, I'm British – if you can't take the mick out of yourself and have a laugh, something is really wrong! In the world of online fitness, the majority of people take themselves extremely seriously the whole time. When I started out, I probably did too, because that's what it seemed like you needed to do to fit in. But as time has gone on, I've just thought, 'To hell with this, I'm just going to be myself.' I've always loved being around people who are happy to make themselves the butt of the joke. Growing up, my younger brother Daniel and I were constantly – literally constantly – in some kind of banter with each other. He has always been really witty and sharp, and we would always be up to no good, cracking jokes and rinsing each other. My friendships are the same, so I guess there has never been much getting away from that. I also think that humour is a good way in. You can tell a lot about someone by what they find funny, and when you're nervous a joke can really help relax things – it's called an ice-breaker for a reason.

I first started posting more jokey content on my extra account @moreoflisafiitt because it felt like it was too 'silly' to be on my main business account. I love a filter, stupid phone effects and some randomness. And I mean real randomness. Romane has always been more serious, and he often doesn't get my jokes, so I find myself laughing by myself. Thank God there are so many weirdos like me out there who get my sense of humour, otherwise I'd probably feel like a loser. I love doing all the funny TikToks and I've slowly started to get Romane involved, though honestly, it's usually just me laughing *at* him. After a while, my funny videos started to get a lot of engagement and attention and some of the best ones went viral. One short clip of me 'slipping' on my diet was reposted by Viola Davis and Amy Schumer (I know, bonkers) and got hundreds of thousands of views. I got all these DMs from American TV shows and people wanting to air my videos, and it just went off. But that's the thing, isn't it? Who isn't looking for a laugh? While I'm definitely not a comedian – can you imagine me having to get up on stage? – I do love bringing comedy into what I do. Just because I take my fitness and business seriously doesn't mean I can't love the lols. I eventually made the decision that I wanted that side of my personality to be part of my main account and 'brand' too, and since I've been incorporating all these funny sketches and videos into my content, I have enjoyed what I do even more.

My followers have responded really well to the light-heartedness, and I think that's because humour helps to connect you to others. I find it so much easier to warm to someone who likes a giggle, especially in the fitness world where everyone is so picture perfect, with blow-dried hair and immaculate make-up, even when lifting weights. I definitely don't do my hair for the gym, and if you've watched any of my content, you'll see I don't look picture-perfect either. After I'd posted my first few videos I got messages saying, 'It's amazing how you really look like you're in pain while you're working out.' For a while I couldn't understand what they meant, then I realised that I was pulling my exercise face – like, you can tell by my face that it's fricking hard! Because the level of vanity is so high on social media and in fitness, it was unusual to see a woman grimacing when she lifted a massive weight. But let's be real – everyone makes faces when they work out, and if they're not doing it on social media, they're either lifting a much lighter weight than they are capable of, or else they're *really* acting (something I am so terrible at). And if you're not making workout faces then you're not working hard enough!

I think humour is an amazing antidote to the self-obsession and narcissism that some of the fitness channels out there promote, and I think it's good to balance the focus on your superficial exterior with something a little more happy-go-lucky. I'm not saying there is anything wrong with taking yourself extremely seriously, it's just that it's not my vibe and never will be. I don't like to be too intense about anything. When you really go in for that 'my lifting schedule is the most important thing that is happening in the world right now' attitude, you can come off as if you really rate yourself. Inevitably, it also becomes all about how you look instead of how you feel, and when your business is to help other people improve their lifestyle and eating habits, it can be off-putting when you seem to be borderline in love with yourself.

Self-love is one thing, and definitely something I've wished I had more of, but I would never want to get caught up in my own hype. Either way, I'm enjoying showing the other side of myself and putting the videos out on my account because I think it really breaks up the more focused workout content. Life can't be all motivation, discipline and body goals – everyone needs a laugh to let off some steam.

Learning what to take seriously – your ambitions, dreams, hard work, mental health and the power of your voice – and what to poke fun at – for me, pretty much everything else – is such an important lesson. No one will take you seriously until you take yourself seriously, and there will always be people out there ready to undermine you, either because it makes them feel better about themselves or because they simply don't have the imagination to envisage your journey. It's normal to have self-doubt, and craving acceptance is natural. That is how we are wired as human beings and one of the reasons that social media 'likes' can be so addictive. I don't know if I will ever be cured of worrying about what other people think of me, but I'm doing my very best to build my own sense of self-belief, regardless of anyone else's opinion. And to my old boss who said I'd never make anything of myself? All I can say is thank you for providing me with the determination to prove you wrong.

STEP FOUR RECAP:

- You are going to be taught so many things about success as you grow up, all of which you will eventually realise are sweeping generalisations. The 'rules' about who can and who can't access success are total rubbish. You don't need to come from a wealthy background or have straight A*s to achieve amazing things in your life. And don't let anyone tell you otherwise.

- If you don't believe in yourself, the sad truth is that no one else will believe in you either. If you want to be taken seriously and for your voice to matter, you have to start taking yourself seriously. Find something you absolutely love doing, invest your time and energy into it, and witness your progress and achievements. That pay-off cannot help but boost your confidence and build your self-esteem.

- You can still achieve while you work on your self-belief. I'm definitely not 'cured' of my insecurities, and I still struggle with all sorts of anxieties related to acceptance and validation. It's ok to be imperfect, and success (especially in a financial sense) won't fix everything. But working to achieve your goals and investing in something you are passionate about is an amazing step in the right direction.

- Take your mental health seriously. It's not just some trend or 'wellness' indulgence. It is something that you should be aware of and make allowances for. If you need to change the way you work to protect your mental health, that should be a priority. Sometimes we are made to feel weak because we make an issue of our struggles; instead we should see it as a strength and work to support each other in finding solutions. If you are not in a good place mentally, you will never be able to achieve everything you hope to.

- On the flip side, it's ok to be silly sometimes! Humour is an amazing release and a way to bond with others. Just because a lot of people on social media take themselves and their fitness schedules very seriously, it doesn't mean you have to. It's meant to be fun and you're meant to enjoy it, otherwise what's the point?!

STEP FOUR TO PHYSICAL STRENGTH: DO YOU NEED SUPPLEMENTS?

It's complicated ...

Romane

The market for dietary supplements is worth over £100 billion globally. That's insane, isn't it? With so many brands advertising so many different powders, pills, bars and drinks, many of which promise to supercharge your fitness journey, it can feel as though there's a lot of pressure to get your supplementation 'right'. And let's be honest, it can also be really expensive. Before I go on – and this is within the context that I do use a range of supplements and Lisa and I have even created our own line of supplements – I just want to say that you have to see supplements as the cherry on the cake. Without a consistent diet and fitness programme,

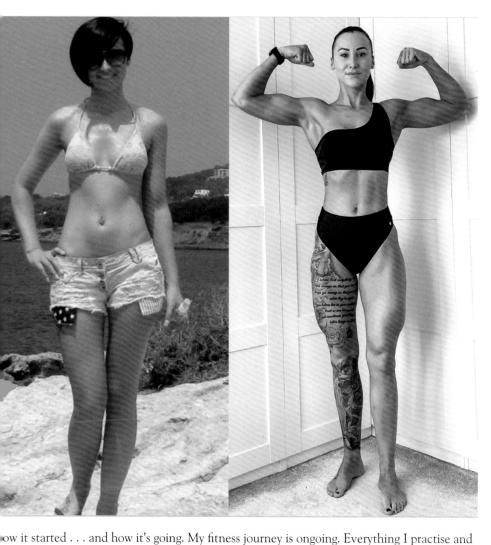

ow it started . . . and how it's going. My fitness journey is ongoing. Everything I practise and
each is about achieving transformational changes to your entire lifestyle, so for me there is
ɔ 'after' in the sense that once you've reached your goal you can't just go back to how you
ere living before. I'm so proud of everything I've achieved so far, but if you want to continue
aping the rewards of the results, you have to remain on this journey forever.

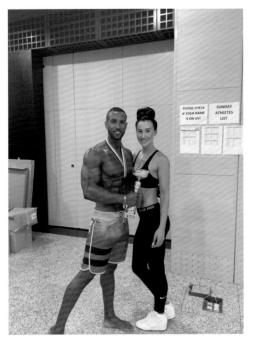

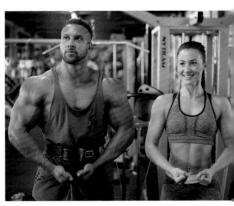

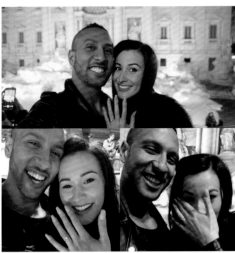

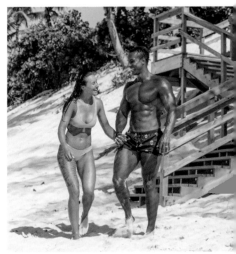

The connection between me and Romane was instant. After three months he proposed to me by the Trevi Fountain in Rome. It's such a cliché to say that when you know, you know – if I'm honest, I think you have to have followed the wrong path to know when something really feels right. But all of it was leading to the most important relationship of my life.

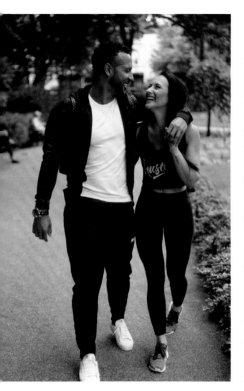

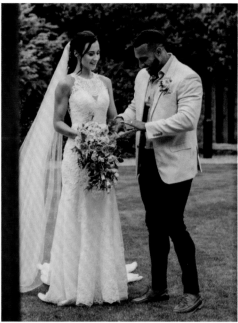

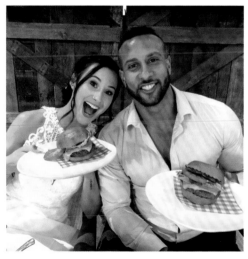

Since the moment we met I have felt at ease with myself when I'm with Romane, and he has been the support structure behind me, building me up as well as providing a cushion to fall back on when things haven't turned out the way I'd hoped. He is an amazing man, who is so driven and so loving, and being around him has inspired me to live a life beyond anything I had ever thought I was capable of.

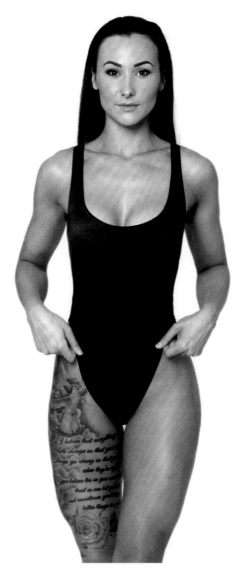

Judging from the comments I get on social media, tattoos really are a love or hate, but I love mine! On my leg I have my favourite quote from Marilyn Monroe, which really resonates with my fitness journey and past relationship.

'I believe that everything happens for a reason. People change so that you can learn to let go, things go wrong so that you can appreciate them when they're right, you believe lies so you eventually learn to trust no one but yourself, and sometimes good things fall apart so better things can fall together.'

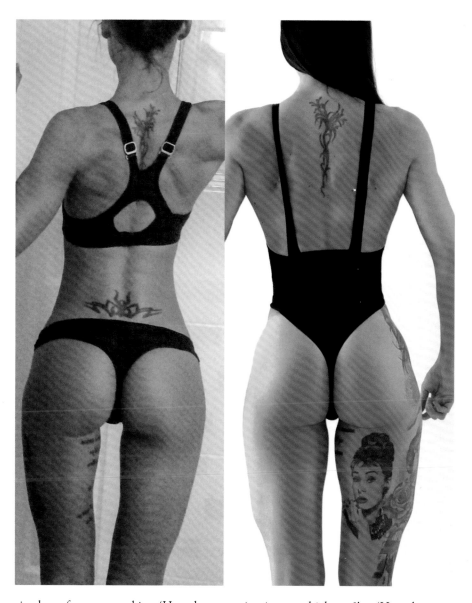

receive lots of messages asking, 'How do you maintain your thigh gap?' or 'How do you get
thigh gap?' A thigh gap is down to BONE STRUCTURE. I don't try to maintain it. It's
omething I have been *very* self-conscious about growing up, due to people staring or making
omments, but I've tried to embrace it and learn to love it (I've personally never seen the
scination with it). You can see how weight training has allowed me to put some meat on in
at area, but in the end it's your body shape that determines whether it is physically possible
r you to have one at all! Most people don't have one and may not be able to achieve one no
atter how much weight they lose, meaning that a thigh gap is not necessarily a healthy goal.
high gap or no thigh gap, we are all beautiful just the way we are!

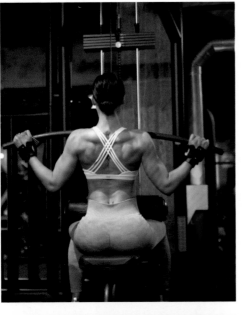

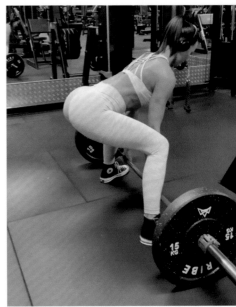

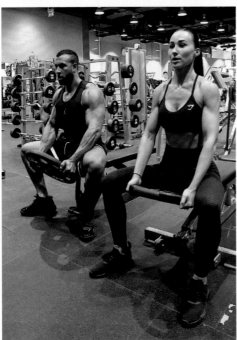

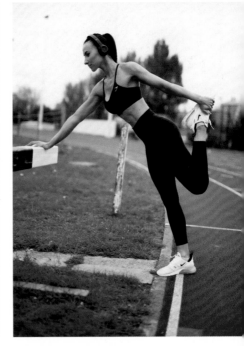

There's a huge misconception that weightlifting is just for bulking, whereas cardio is for your heart and general health. The fact is, the two are far more connected than we have been led to believe. There is even research that suggests weightlifting is *better* than cardio for guarding against heart disease. That's why I think it's so important that women are encouraged to get into the weight room and find the balance that works for them.

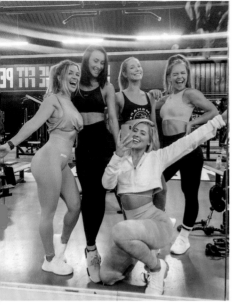

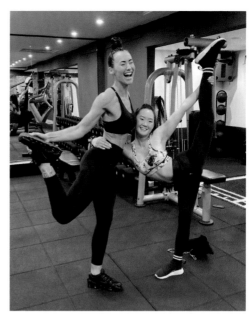

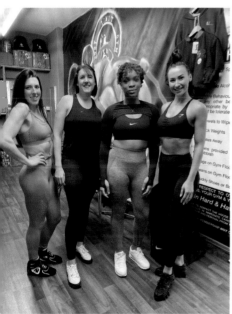

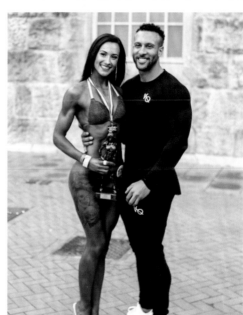

he people around you have a huge impact on your happiness and quality of life. Negativity nd toxicity can be catastrophic for your self-esteem and confidence, so it's worth being really onest with yourself about your relationships and whether individuals are supporting you or olding you back.

raining with someone who can be that cheerleader for you, whether it's a friend, partner or T, is really amazing for helping to push you to the next stage and combat any lack of elf-belief. While I also enjoy training on my own, it's never quite as fun as when we train gether.

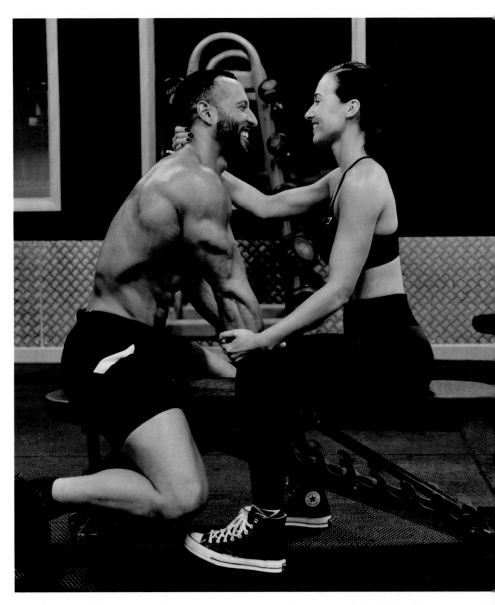

Living strong is a holistic choice, which impacts every area of your life. If you want to continue to reap the rewards of your mental and physical strength, you have to continue to invest in them. Remember, you can do amazing things. You just have to take the first step.

supplements aren't going to do much. They won't do you any harm, but they're certainly not going to transform your body unless you change the rest of your lifestyle. So, they are definitely not something to be losing sleep over.

What supplements *can* do is help you to reach your overall goals and save you a lot of time, making your life much more convenient. Which in our busy lives today, is really valuable. Nearly all supplements will have a benefit, but if something doesn't agree with you, just stop taking it. Missing a day of protein or your multivitamins is not going to scupper your chances of reaching your potential, but there is no doubt that supplements can really support your journey, so it's worth considering your options and giving them a go.

It's probably best to start by looking at the range of products out there and understanding what is and isn't worth your money and time. Most supplements offer you micronutrients, but it's a macronutrient – protein – which is the big daddy of supplements, and both Lisa and I take some kind of protein supplement every day. As I mentioned earlier, it is possible to get all the protein your need for hypertrophy through your diet (especially if you have a lower body weight), but keeping that protein level topped up all day long (as you can't store excess protein) can sometimes be a challenge, and that's where supplements come in. Unless you choose a vegan protein (which is most often made from pea, hemp, brown rice or soy protein), your protein source will likely be from whey or casein protein from milk. Working out which protein is best can become overcomplicated. While we were working on our own protein supplement, we tried so many varieties, and the truth is that most are very similar, with broadly similar ratios of protein to calorie/carb/fat, though one might have maybe half a gram more sugar than another. The margins are pretty small. What you will probably find, however, is that some proteins are harder on your gut than others, and some might make you feel bloated, which is obviously not what you want.

There are three general options: a simple protein concentrate, which is made by extracting protein from milk using heat and acids or enzymes, and will typically consist of 60–80 per cent protein, with the remaining 20–40 per cent made up of carbs and fats (something you do need to take into account when working out your overall calorie and macro intake). There are also protein isolates, which go through an additional filtering process to remove more fat and carbs, creating an even more concentrated protein source – around 90–95 per cent. The final option is protein hydrolysate, which goes through even more heating, with additional acids and enzymes breaking down the bonds between the amino acids. Hydrolysates are therefore easier for the body and your muscles to absorb, which is why Lisa and I decided to go with them for our own protein supplement. Hydrolysates also appear to raise insulin levels more than other forms of protein, at least in the case of whey protein. This can enhance muscle growth following exercise (the greater the insulin response, the greater the muscle protein growth after resistance training).

While isolates and hydrolysates are more expensive, when we were creating our supplements we wanted to make the very best, which we could stand behind 100 per cent. However, if you can't afford more than the basic protein concentrate, you will still get great benefits from the simpler option. What you're looking for is a powder that offers 25g of protein per scoop. Lisa has 25g of protein per shake (we like ours with porridge oats and serve it cold, which people always think is super-strange; there are no health benefits to this – it's just our preference!) and I have 50g. Lisa will have one shake a day on top of her usual dietary protein intake, and I'll generally have two over the course of a day. The most beneficial time to drink a shake is post-workout, so as soon as you've finished training, ensure you've got a protein source right there to hand. If you think it might take you an hour to get showered, changed and home, it's really useful to grab a shake straight away, to make sure the protein is topped up and ready to do its work after you've trained.

If you look on the shelves of a health or fitness store, you will also see amino acid supplements (amino acids are the building blocks of proteins). BCAAs (three branched-chain essential amino acids: leucine, isoleucine and valine) and EAAs (essential amino acids – the full nine: leucine, isoleucine, valine, histidine, lysine, methionine, phenylalanine, threonine and tryptophan – don't worry, there isn't a test at the end!) are the two main varieties you will see widely available. If you have your protein intake under control, you will have all of these micronutrients ready to go, but the benefit of these amino acid supplements is that unlike protein powders, they don't have any calories at all. So why doesn't everyone just ditch the protein and take amino acids instead? Well, protein in the form of whey is a complete protein source, offering the body the perfect package of amino acids in exactly the right amounts for muscle building. Amino acids just don't satisfy daily protein demands, and if you take too many of one it can cause a metabolic imbalance – so if you take too much leucine, for example, you'll have an imbalance of the other amino acids. Research has also shown that amino acid supplements alone are not enough to promote muscle growth, however a systematic study has shown that additional amino acid supplementation *can* help repair low-level muscle damage. If it's a choice between the two, go protein all the way, but that doesn't mean there isn't value to amino acid supplements too.

The other popular macronutrient supplement is the mass gainer, and this is the only one I'd recommend you avoid, because it's a total rip-off. As a teenager, I was desperate to gain weight, and I spent all my pocket money on absolutely rubbish mass gainer powders. Most of the gym bros out there have tried a mass gainer at some point – five shovel scoops of this disgusting stuff, at 2,000 calories a shake, as thick as ice cream so you can barely drink it. Women seem much less likely to try them (probably because of the huge calorie level). The truth is that they cost more than food, are pumped with so much rubbish and just make you gain body fat. The body just cannot use all those calories. If you need to increase your calorie intake, just add some more oats to your shaker with whey, or top up with some pure nut butter – it's so much more delicious and a fraction of the price.

Creatine is another very popular supplement, and rightly so because it can have a really marked impact on your performance. As a nutrient, it's similar to amino acids (your body makes it from arginine and glycine), and 95 per cent of it is stored in the muscles as phosphocreatine, which helps your body produce a high-energy molecule called adenosine triphosphate (ATP). And when you have more ATP, your body performs better during exercise, simple as that. Everyone who trains should probably take creatine, because it's good value and extremely effective for building muscle and power. We actually don't take it because it really affected Lisa's skin – she found that it created little popping blisters across her back, which cleared up as soon as she stopped taking the tablets. You do have to be careful with creatine: in my younger days I overdid it during what's marketed as the 'loading phase', when you go heavy with your intake. Too much creatine can overload the kidneys and make you feel really weak and fatigued. It's also been proven that you don't need to tank it to load at the beginning of use as is sometimes advised and if you just have one scoop a day for a longer period, it has the same benefits.

As for other micronutrients, I do take a lot of vitamin and mineral supplements, including a high-quality multivitamin, cod liver oil and turmeric. I'd also really recommend trying glucosamine if you've ever experienced any joint-related injuries (it's found in cartilage, the cushion to all of our joints) and supplements are either harvested from shellfish or made in a lab.

For all supplements, make sure you read the full labelling and consult a doctor if you have any specific conditions that might be complicated by a dietary supplement – often people forget that these powders and pills are just the same as wholefoods in that sense.

Now I'm going to be moderately controversial here and add one more supplement into the mix: caffeine. Before I go any further, I want to clarify that I don't support the use of caffeine to keep you awake. If you are exhausted because you aren't getting enough sleep, you should never use caffeine to help get you to the gym. Always listen to your body. But if you are in good health and generally have good energy levels, but perhaps need that little pick-me-up before you head to the weight room to push your performance, I think there is definitely a place for caffeine. A good caffeine supplement helps me to train harder for longer and I enjoy it a lot more. Both Lisa and I have had our best stretches of training and made the most improvements when we've been using a good caffeine supplement. It's like you get to the gym and feel like you don't want to leave. I wouldn't say that you have a perceptible buzz or that you feel wired, it's more that you suddenly notice you've done all of these sets and exercises, but you feel like you can keep going.

Caffeine is usually sold as a pre-workout powder or drink, though you might find some people recommending a shot of espresso twenty minutes before hitting the gym. As with everything, it's what works best for you that matters. For me, finding a good caffeine supplement has often meant the difference between getting the work done and not getting the work done. It's the difference between sacking it off and nailing it. I would definitely caution against overusing caffeine, especially if you are a big coffee drinker anyway; you do not want to keep chasing that first high you got from a great pre-workout, progressively adding more and more, because too much caffeine can perpetuate anxiety, stop you sleeping properly, and in some cases even lead to high blood pressure and migraines. So don't be silly about it – read the health advice and take it seriously.

Coming back to what I said right at the top of this chapter, my main message is that you have to get your diet working for you. So many people will sign up to the gym and immediately buy fourteen expensive, fancy supplements, and that is not what we're advocating. First, get your meals right, then go from there. Experiment with supplements, and don't just focus on the impact on your performance, but look at how they affect your skin and tummy, too. They have to offer a holistic benefit to your life, as health and happiness are the ultimate goals. And finally, don't ever think about buying a mass gainer – trust me, you'll regret it.

STEP FIVE TO MENTAL STRENGTH:
STOP FAKING IT 'TIL YOU MAKE IT

Put the work in instead

If there's one phrase that encapsulates Instagram culture, it's 'fake it 'til you make it'. You hear people saying it all the time, up and down the country, almost like an anthem. The problem is that I think the whole idea of faking anything is ultimately detrimental for your mental health. So many people in my generation have issues with imposter syndrome and anxiety, and I feel like so much of that comes from the pressure to pretend that you can do something – or that you are something – when you can't or you're not. The underlying reason to fake it 'til you make it is to speed up your progress in some area of your life. Everyone is in such a rush to get to the top that they want to fast-forward through earning their spurs, which was once seen as

162

necessary to be able to reach any goal. I'm not saying don't put on a great outfit for an interview or prepare for a presentation to impress your boss. We all have to put a bit of a public face on, even when we're actually really nervous, and I suppose that could be seen as a bit of fakery. But attempting to leapfrog over the weeks, months and years of experience that can give you *true* confidence and self-belief is just shooting yourself in the foot ultimately, and I think more people need to come out and say that.

Not being able to do something which I've said I could, is probably my worst nightmare and I know a lot of other people feel the same way. It's enough to bring me out in a cold sweat. Even when I feel deeply confident about my ability to do something, I still don't like being put on the spot, so imagine what it would feel like if you really didn't know what you were talking about! The stress would just be too much for me. But when you're encouraged by everyone to basically wing it or learn 'on the job', you can start to feel like you're missing a trick or at least falling way behind other people by doing things the old-fashioned way. I just want to say that if you're like me, hold out, take your time and you'll make it without ever having to cope with the pressures of faking it.

What weightlifting has taught me is the value of long-term investment in achieving all of my goals. You can't build muscle overnight – it takes dedication, consistency and time. You can't fake it. Even if you were to take steroids, you still have to do the work. You have to turn up and make it happen day after day. There are no results without work, and that philosophy should translate to all areas of our lives. The value of experience needs to be re-established as aspirational; we have all got a bit too interested in flash in the pan.

In the fitness world on Instagram, the fake it 'til you make it message is rife. There is absolutely nothing to stop anyone setting up an account, saying they are a fitness professional and selling you something based on the way their body looks. As we've discussed, there's such a vast genetic variation out there that one person might be able to make their body look amazing with relatively little effort. When you factor in photographic angles and the editing software available – including video photoshopping – there is the potential for some serious fakery. Like PT catfishing! This is obviously an extreme example, but this kind of deception is on a spectrum and a lot of people are playing the game to a lesser or greater extent.

What I would say is that in weightlifting and fitness in general, there is no substitute for experience. One issue we have is that the education system prioritises qualifications over everything. While that might be appropriate if you're going to be a doctor or scientist, for many other jobs experience is so much more valuable than anything you can gain from a textbook. Qualifications are all good, but in my industry they're little more than a piece of paper.

Before I met Romane, I had decided to do a personal training course, because I was so enjoying weightlifting and felt like I could have a future working as a PT. The appeal was centred around the idea that I knew I could help other people, and I just loved being in the gym, so I wanted to find a way to make it part of my working life. It felt like a good idea to do some kind of course, at least as a starting point, because if you want to be taken seriously and be treated as a legitimate professional, you need a qualification, right? When I moved to Bristol with Romane, I found a course just down the road and I started to build the foundations of my knowledge of the body. I'm not going to lie, it was really hard – I was so new to it all, and I had no background in that area. I'm also not overly academic and I do struggle in more traditional learning environments, but I managed to pass everything on the course. From a practical perspective, however, so many of the movements we were assessed on were very basic, and when I look at my form generally back then, it was terrible! There are very few advanced techniques included in PT training courses – no deadlifts or many of the movements that I now use and teach on a daily basis. It's mainly just bicep curls, sitting on the leg extension machine, and doing tricep dips, so when it came to what I actually needed to transform my own body, the knowledge I gained was pretty limited.

To be completely frank, I would not have been able to go straight into personal training after finishing the course. Absolutely no way! We have been led to believe that once you've passed the test and got the piece of paper – bang, you're done. Um, no. Just because I had a qualification, I was not qualified to give anyone advice. I didn't have the experience, even in my own body, and while I could have gone out there, all guns blazing, telling people that I was a 'fully qualified PT', I would have been totally faking it, which is just not my style. I'm never really sure how people manage to pull this off in fitness, because how do you even know what to say to your clients? I would feel so terrible inside, knowing that I was almost lying to people. Especially when it's something so important – people's health – that you are influencing. If you end up doing a certain exercise in the wrong way, you could really hurt someone. Or if you give flawed nutritional advice, you might cause people to be undernourished, and there are so many health risks there.

It's not just the technique and form that is important for teaching, it's knowing how to put training plans together for different goals and understanding how different bodies respond to different exercises. Most of that is trial and error informed by what you've experienced with your own body and what you've learned from others around you over time. Back in the day, I wouldn't have had a clue, but over the years you do your own research, test it out in the gym and build up a huge bank of knowledge. Without experience, the theories are pretty empty, and when you are talking about something like fitness which is so physical, there is just no replacement for actually doing it. That's what truly counts. The past six years have taught me everything I could ever need to know, and I've learned so much more than I did on my course.

As we decided to take our business online right from the get-go, I didn't have any in-gym PT'ing experience. But if I were to decide to become a PT now – and who knows, I might end up doing that one day – I would be so secure in myself and have so much confidence because of the thousands of people I have trained and worked with over this time.

I know I have been really fortunate, because I've also had the opportunity to learn from incredible competitors and have gained so much knowledge from Romane and his peers. Together we've travelled the world and trained with other amazing IFBB professional bodybuilders, which has been an amazing experience for me. Almost from the beginning of my journey, I was introduced to advanced techniques. At the start, that was pretty daunting, because I was still on a bit of a learning curve and a lot of the methods bodybuilders used were not taught generally or even covered on social media. It gave me such an incredible insight right out of the gate and meant that I used advanced and highly targeted techniques to build the foundations of the body I have today. Now I'm seeing so many more people talking about these kinds of techniques, because they're becoming more mainstream. The more people talk about something, the more people learn from each other, and so it snowballs, which is really cool and I love that I'm a part of spreading that knowledge, gained from years of experience, and helping so many people access information which could help them.

As for my career in social media, for me trust is everything. It helps that I'd never be able to wangle my through anything. Or pull the wool over anyone's eyes anyway. I am the world's worst liar, so it's not really a choice for me. I was very much raised to know that honesty is the best policy, and the fear of being caught out in a lie or even a minor deception is enough to keep me honest for life. When it comes to my associations with other businesses or developing my own products, I've always held true to the belief that you have to put the work in. Both Romane and I like to be really straightforward and never big up anything we don't think is that great. We're not over the top people, and we're not exaggerators. Everyone has that friend, don't they! But when it comes to our business, whenever we bring out products, we have to truly believe in them.

If we were working with 100 different brands, it would be hard for people to believe that every single one of them was 100 per cent amazing, right? I've always preferred to wait until the right collaborations came along, and so I haven't signed with every brand out there. Generally, I would prefer to not take the money for a partnership and instead take my time to develop my own products which I am fully accountable for. If an amazing brand comes to me with an offer which I feel is really the very best, and I know I wouldn't be able to do any better myself, then great. But if I can't talk about a product with passion and be able to convey that it's something I truly believe in, I can't support it. On top of hard work, transparency is so important. At the end of the day, people are spending their hard-earned money here and I know from experience how hard money is to make. So we want to make sure that our products are the best they can be and that we are offering our community the best value we possibly can.

That does mean we have to be really patient with the pace of what we put out there though, which obviously flies in the face of the 'get rich quick', 'fake it 'til you make it' culture. Sometimes Romane and I feel like we come from a different time than a lot of the people we see on social media, because our projects are often years in the making, when a twelve-week turnaround seems to be the norm for others. We do sometimes wonder why we are so slow comparatively, but time and time again it's proven to be the right path. Take the case of our supplements line. We have been talking about it for three or four years, but it really took shape about two years ago. The starting point was that I could never find a protein powder that agreed with my tummy. My situation was not unusual – so many people complain about bloating with protein powders, and for me, every time I had a shake, my tummy would churn and sound really funny. In turn that would make me feel sluggish and not very nice at all. So we started to delve into it and began sampling lots and lots of different options to try to find something which was easier on my digestive system.

The more we looked into it, the more we knew we wanted to go with a hydrolysed protein (see Step Four to Physical Strength) as it's a lot easier for the body to digest than standard whey protein. I wanted to test it for a few months to make sure that it continued to agree with me and to ensure it was truly effective for what we wanted it to do, i.e. support gains and maintenance. We did so much sampling, and there was so much back and forth, so we could be certain it would work for digestion not just once, but thirty times. Knowing we had full control over every element of the process made me feel so confident about what we were doing. Completing the full diligence and personally feeling the effects of products on our own bodies was non-negotiable for us, but it's worth understanding that not everyone who puts their name to a product goes through such a rigorous process. There is no law against me giving my name to a third-party company, never even trying a product and then promoting it through my Instagram. That's a really scary thought for me, but it is the reality of how a lot of business deals go in the online fitness world and beyond.

Another reason for launching our own supplement range was because people were always asking us what we supplemented with, and I just didn't feel comfortable telling people to take something that I wasn't completely happy with. But now we've built this collection of stripped-back basics, I do feel confident sharing it. Because my lord, we did the work! Of course, there is always the chance that a supplement won't agree with you as we are all made differently and, especially with whey, there can be issues of dairy intolerance and sensitivity. But what we have put together should agree with the majority of people, and that is such a feeling of achievement. I'm particularly proud of the vegan protein, because everything else out there is pretty disgusting and ours tastes really good – so much effort went into that! Right now, the range includes bars, energy drinks, protein, a pre-workout and EAAs, so it's just the core requirements, and we will continue testing and adding more over time where we feel we can make a difference.

I hope my story helps anyone struggling in school or college to realise that they can end up being so good at so many things, even if they aren't an A* student. I really wish schools helped kids understand the value of experience and didn't just focus on exams and GCSEs, as I do believe it would help so many people with their confidence. I wish somebody had told me – no one ever said take your time, learn and hone your craft, build your confidence and experience over time and you will fly. My advice to anyone thinking about a particular course or career path would be to get at least some experience before you sign up and pay. The benefit of that is that you will be able to see if you actually like something instead of just liking the idea of something. When I look back to my hairdressing and all the time and energy I invested into my qualifications, I do feel like it was a bit of a waste. In that instance, it was as much about feeling that my options were limited, but it's crazy to think how much I went through with my training now as I've never used the qualifications once.

If someone were to ask me for advice when starting a career in fitness, the first thing I would say is to join a gym. Start working with your own body. Book a few PT sessions and learn the basics, and at the same time ask your trainer about the realities of their job and what they love and hate about it. This will help you decide if it's something you want to do, and can also give you that bit of knowledge and provide you with the confidence to take the next step. The first-day-at-school feeling is so hard, but having a bit of know-how really does make it less intimidating. If you're passionate about something and you love it, gaining experience in that field won't feel like a chore. And it's got to be better than spending time and effort on something then realising it's just not for you. I also think getting real life experience in an industry is really humbling because it makes you understand how much you don't know, as well as giving you respect for the professionals who are ahead of you in their careers. If you have experience, you don't just think you're top of the tree because you passed an exam, and you have the chance to find mentors and build a community of people around you who can help you grow.

Going into anything blind is really overwhelming. In the digital age, it's tempting to think that you can find

173

everything you need to know on the internet, and of course we all use Google when we are learning. But you have to be so careful. Aside from the rampant misinformation out there, the world is incredibly opinionated and some people express their opinions as if they're set in stone, when in reality there's a lot of grey areas and a lot of information about the body is contested. There just haven't been enough studies on the various ways the body functions to draw 100 per cent conclusions on certain elements. The physical steps in this book are all based on the most up-to-date research, but things change all the time, and new discoveries shift the way we view something. Of course, Romane also has two decades of experience to ground his advice, which is worth so much.

Even if you manage to dodge the fake news, you may encounter two people who hold the exact opposite beliefs about calories, say, or the best form for a deadlift. And without experience, it's almost impossible to tell which 'side' is right as the 'experts' always sound very convincing. Usually, both sides are partly right and the arguments are just a waste of time and energy. Why no one can say, 'Some people do things this way, while other people do things that way and both have value,' I don't know. I suppose that's not the atmosphere of social media. But the righteousness out there, the 'You're doing it wrong, this is the right way, and I'm the one that knows best' attitude can be really confusing and intimidating if you don't have confidence in your own knowledge.

I always say to our app community that as long as you're not creating the potential for injury, there is value in any movement. For example, when it comes to squats, the internet will make you believe there is one single right way to do them, which will fast-track you to the perfect bum, and everything else is a waste of time. That is just so wrong. There isn't just one way to do squats – it's whatever fits your body's anatomy. All of our joints are different, we are all working with different calf elasticity and ankle mobility. Instead, the advice should be to play around with it, because what might work for someone else won't work for your body make-up. The problem is that things can get so heated that even I occasionally find I'm second-guessing myself, but it's my experience that brings me back to my confidence in what I'm doing and what I know.

As long as your movement isn't going to cause an injury, how you do it is your business. Yes, there are optimum ways to target certain muscles and I will always explain that in my guidance, but the whole idea of the one-and-only method for progress is such rubbish. It's worth noting that different areas of the fitness world have different ways of doing things anyway. A few years ago, at the beginning of my journey, I posted a video of me doing a cable row and some guy made a comment on my form. My form was that I stretched out and then pulled back in, which is the body-building way of doing it. He obviously hadn't encountered that before and so he unloaded his criticisms publicly. It really upset me at the time because I questioned myself straight away. I was like oh my God, I'm going to be one of those PTs where people say, 'that PT needs a PT' kind of thing. I was still very new to everything and trying to learn and I just thought, 'He's right, I'm terrible at this, I shouldn't be posting.' But if someone said that to me now, I'd be like, 'Nah, let me tell you!' I know what I know. What I find so mind-boggling is that there are people out there who are maybe only 10 per cent sure of what they know, but they're prepared to unleash on other people as if they were the God of all gyms. People do love to try and tell you that you're wrong. I find it's often guys who feel like they need to edu-cate you as a woman in the industry. But you only have to look to see that there is a Pilates way of doing a sit-up, a yoga way of doing a sit-up, a bodybuilding way of doing a sit-up, and guess what? They're all sit-ups and they all tone your abs.

My biggest takeaway from my fitness journey is how powerful experience can be. The confidence I feel inside because of what I've learned as much as what I've achieved physically is so strong that sometimes I can't believe it. And when you back yourself so completely in an area of your life, it's catching. Because I know my stuff in the gym, I feel more confident in other areas of my life. That doesn't mean I suddenly think I'm an expert in everything – in fact it's the opposite. I now have so much respect for professionals in any field because I know what it takes to gain that kind of knowledge and build those skills.

So don't try to fake it 'til you make it. Instead, do the work, put in the time and earn your spurs. Then you won't be an imposter, you'll be an expert who knows exactly what you're claiming to know, and that's true confidence.

STEP FIVE RECAP:

- We live in an era when you're often encouraged to over-state your skills and abilities. For so many of us even thinking about saying you can do something before you've even tested yourself is horrendously anxiety-inducing. Never feel foolish for taking your time, building your experience, and then going out into the world with your abilities and services. It will pay off in the long run and spare you countless sleepless nights.
- It feels like we have forgotten and diminished the value of experience. Starting in school we're often made to believe that exams, qualifications and certificates are seen

as more important than hands-on, 'real-life' experience. There's sometimes a snobbery around it, with people more likely to believe a teenager who has a certificate from a three-day course than a veteran who has been training ad hoc for ten years without any formal education. That way of thinking is so backward because you can't fake or make any kind of substitute for experience. That's the gold standard in so many fields, including fitness.

- Social media can be the wild west, especially when it comes to selling products. Be wary of creators who put their names to anything and everything, or seem to be bringing out collections and ranges every other week. Full oversight takes time and investment, whereas signing a contract to use your name for something takes seconds.

- Experience has provided me with the confidence needed to stand my ground in a really contentious environment. When you work in an industry where there are lots of opinions and egos, and a lot of people who believe their methods and ways of doing things are the best, establishing your own beliefs and holding your own is so vital to having the self-belief to go out there and do things your way.

- Don't feel like the chancers are leaving you for dust, because their success is built on sand. That might sound like something your mum would say, but it's just realistic.

When you're young it can be really hard to be patient because you want to get the finish line yesterday. But building up your experience, body and wisdom over time will create a deep sense of confidence, which will serve you so much better in the long run. Plus, you won't have to be constantly looking your shoulder, worrying that someone is going to find you out!

STEP FIVE TO PHYSICAL STRENGTH: THE POWER OF HYDRATION

Why simple H_2O is the best anabolic you've never heard of

Romane

For anyone looking to dramatically improve the way they look and feel without totally upending their current lifestyle, I always give the same simple advice: drink more water. Even if you're not ready to follow every other step in this book, making sure you are properly hydrated is an incredible first goal, which everyone can achieve on the trek up that mountain. Haven't made it to the gym? Not done fantastic with the diet? Tomorrow is another day. Have a couple of glasses of water and know that you're giving your body all the hydration it needs. As for gains, well, hypertrophy ain't happening without hydration, so it's time to buy a water bottle, keep it full and learn to drink properly.

That might sound like really basic advice, but in all seriousness, the vast majority of people don't drink enough water on a daily basis to thrive and be their best selves, both physically and mentally. For those of us privileged enough to live in an environment where water is plentiful and available at the turn of a tap, it's absolutely crazy.

Most of us know that water is important, but when it comes to the why, you might be a little fuzzy. Aside from the fact that water makes up 60 per cent of our body, 73 per cent of our brain and heart and 83 per cent of our lungs, every cell in the body uses water. You can't survive without water for more than a few days because innumerable processes just can't happen without sufficient water supply. Your blood is about 92 per cent water, and without blood, oxygen can't be carried around the body, and without oxygen, your cells will die. Water keeps your temperature stable, it's needed to digest your food, and to get rid of it too.

As for your muscles, we are talking about 79 per cent water. While we all chat about proteins and supplements, water is the biggest anabolic agent out there. It plays a key part in muscle growth because it's what transports the nutrients – protein's amino acid blocks and glycogen – to the tissues to repair the myofibrils torn by lifting weights. The more water you drink, the greater the blood volume and flow to the muscles. You can tell when you're sufficiently hydrated while training because you feel that 'pump' sensation as your muscles are filled with nutrient-rich blood, ready to set about repairing things. Equally, you know when you're dehydrated because your muscles will look comparatively empty and flat.

You might wonder what the actual impact of dehydration might be on your results, and you'd be forgiven for thinking it couldn't be that big a deal, because water just doesn't get much hype or press (probably because it's free and no one can make much money out of it). But studies have shown that even being moderately dehydrated (about 3 per cent of your body weight) can have a negative impact on your ability to train as well as your ability to build muscle. It appears that for anaerobic exercises (which break down glucose without using oxygen; generally high-intensity activities for short periods) like weightlifting, performance is particularly impaired by dehydration. Endurance has been shown to be reduced by up to 8 per cent and muscle strength by 5 per cent – and this is just with moderate dehydration. Even 1.5 per cent dehydration has been shown to decrease the muscle strength of one rep – and when your rep strength or count is hit, you aren't going to be growing muscle in the same strength or size and your workout just isn't going to be that effective. It's such a simple thing and yet it has the power to undermine your potential for growth.

Aside from muscle growth, water also plays a role in fat loss, so if one of your body goals is to reduce body fat, it's an invaluable addition to your daily routine. Water is essential for burning fat from food and drink, as well as from stored fat through the process of lipolysis – breaking down those triglycerides into usable energy. Water also takes up space in the stomach, which leads to a feeling of fullness that may stop you reaching for the biscuit tin, especially if you consume it with food, or in the form of soup, for example. Whenever my clients say they're finding themselves hungry between meals, I always tell them to check in with their hydration, as often we think we're hungry when we're actually thirsty. Topping up your liquid first is the best way to deal with hunger pangs – if you're still peckish twenty minutes later, you know your body is actually hungry, because water on its own will pass pretty quickly through your stomach.

Chronic mild dehydration has been associated with obesity, diabetes, cancer and cardiovascular disease. But on a less doomsday level, dehydration can absolutely lessen your quality of life on a day-to-day basis. The number of people who have got to a place where they think it's normal to trudge through their day feeling lethargic, with a near constant headache, on the edge of moodiness is truly mind-blowing. Mild dehydration has been shown to impact short-term memory, alertness, concentration and impair your motor skills. The scientific term is 'general malaise', which means feeling ill and despondent. It literally sucks you dry all day long and that sucks. You deserve so much better than that.

After reading this I really hope your next question is: how do I make sure I'm never dehydrated again?! Well, you're obviously going to live and escaping mild hydration every single day for the rest of your life is probably going to be impossible, especially if you live in a hot climate. In fact, if you work outdoors or exercise in the heat, you could lose up to 10 litres of water in sweat, so the focus has to be on fluid replacement. Getting used to carrying water with you at all times is a great choice for your health. It may mean you have to invest in a new bag as well as a water bottle to make sure you always have it with you and certainly never, ever begin a workout before you've fully hydrated yourself.

As a rule of thumb, about 2 litres of water a day for women and 3 litres of water a day for men should keep you covered without going too far. Because you *can* go too far when it comes to water – overhydration can lead to sodium dilution in the blood, which at its worse can lead to heart failure, so think more about sipping water throughout the day rather than chugging six bottles all at once. And remember that you can get water from food too, especially plant-based foods. In general, we get about 20 per cent of our water from our food, and if you stack up the cucumbers, celery and tomatoes in there, you have a great water source without adding another glass to your routine.

While our bodies have complex, sophisticated ways of maintaining water concentration in the blood, with thirst signals being the most obvious, nutritional scientists have found that the body can lose 1–2 per cent of its weight before that craving for liquid kicks in, and that amount can be enough to have an impact on your body's function. There is still a place for thirst as a signal, but it's better to keep your hydration levels ticking over before you feel parched – we like to be sure we have enough protein in our diet with a slight surplus, and we do the same with water.

I've hydrated since I can remember, but I also sweat a lot. In fact, while I'm in the gym, it's impossible for me to keep up with my water loss, so I have to ensure I continue to hydrate after I leave to make sure I replace everything lost through training. For Lisa, it's almost the opposite. Before she got into fitness, she hardly drank anything. Her mum, who was a nurse, was always telling her to drink to support her kidneys and renal system, and when she started her classes, she changed things up with a big bottle at her desk every day.

Now she is just like me, and if she doesn't hydrate properly, she feels it so quickly. Both of us would say that we now absolutely hate to feel dehydrated, and we can identify it immediately. It will generally happen over the space of three or four hours, and the first sign for me at least is grogginess and fatigue. Aside from that you'll notice that your urine is a darker colour or you wee a lot less, and you might even find that those headaches turn into migraines. You could feel lightheaded or dizzy and your lips, eyes and mouth might feel uncomfortably dry. The best thing about water is that as soon as you start drinking, all of these symptoms will go into reverse.

As mentioned before, exercising while dehydrated is absolutely not going to lead to the most effective workout or help you reach your potential. And of course, it will only dehydrate you more. Aside from always carrying water with you, it's great to create a habit and rhythm around it: Pre-hydrate – Exercise – Rehydrate – Repeat. That means you should arrive at the mat hydrated, but also replenish your water reserves throughout a workout session to ensure your body is in the optimum state. If you are training at a high level, it might also be worth trying a sports drink to help replace any salts and electrolytes that are lost through sweat, but always check the label as you'll find many of these drinks are pumped full of sugar, which would have an impact on your overall calorie intake. That's definitely something to take into account if you're substituting water with juice, smoothies or fizzy drinks – while they will of course have an impact on your daily fluid intake, they also have additional kcals which could undermine your overall goals. Water (with its 0 kcals) remains the best option for hydration. Get your water intake right and you will not only see progress in the gym, but you'll find that your general health and wellbeing are improved in every other aspect of your life too. What's not to love about that?

STEP SIX TO MENTAL STRENGTH:
GREAT EXPECTATIONS

How to leave behind other people's ideas of who you are

Back in my parents' day, most people were meant to follow a fairly similar path: do the same things around the same time and live the same kind of life. But today many of us have ended up in jobs our parents couldn't have even imagined, and we've met people, even our partners, through our phones in a way that would have seemed alien even a decade ago. We've built businesses and travelled widely, meeting and encountering different cultures and experiences, all of which enriches our understanding of the world. But for some reason, it's like we still can't shake all the rules of the old world, and the expectations of how our lives will turn out continue to be there in the background. Are they engaged? Are they getting married? Are they pregnant? How much is their house worth? You hear the phrase 2.4 children or for a woman, hear the ages of 30, 35 or 40 and you have some kind of idea in your mind about where you are meant to be or what you are meant to have achieved, and that does have an impact on how you feel about your life.

Social media has added a whole new layer to those expectations. We now have ideas about what our homes should look like, how many luxury holidays we should go on, what car we should be driving. And it's not only a pressure we put on ourselves; there are also expectations from other people about what we should be doing. For me, as a married thirty-two-year-old on social media, the focus, pretty much every day, is on when I'm going to get pregnant. Now don't get me wrong, I really want a family – Romane and I are so looking forward to that journey, and it's definitely on our minds more than it has ever been before. But seriously, you have no idea how often I'm asked about it. As soon as Romane and I got engaged, the baby question started, and it hasn't stopped since. People ask us wherever we go, in person, in comments and DMs, on TikTok, Facebook and Instagram, or say, 'It'll be you guys next ... ' Well, maybe. I don't know. Soon, perhaps.

I absolutely know it comes most often from a place of love and because people are so excited for us to build a family, but sometimes it's just a bit mind-boggling. There have been numerous occasions when I've posted a teaser on my stories about an announcement coming. I'll say that it's something we've been working so hard on and it will feature a picture of us both looking strong. That same day, I will also have posted pictures of myself training in a crop top and leggings, which I would have thought would indicate that it's nothing to do with me being pregnant. Minimum 90 per cent of the responses and DMs will be asking me if I'm pregnant. It's all 'baby, baby, baby'. And even when I haven't mentioned any particular news, I'll also get messages saying that I *look like* I'm pregnant. It gets to the stage where other people's expectations start to actually influence you – if so many people are expecting me to be pregnant, should I be thinking about it too? And there is something very weird about that, but as a woman on social media, I don't seem to be able to avoid it.

I'm using this example because I think that in many ways, there is still a lot of pressure on women to conform to certain ideas of how they should live their lives, and I think we should all be aware of those pressures so we can try and stand aside from them when we make our choices, to ensure we're doing things that we actually want to do.

But seeing as this is my book and I'm being honest with you, I'm happy to share my thoughts on the baby question.

I definitely used to be really intimidated and scared about the idea of getting pregnant, because my body is my profession and it's what our business is based on. But recently – and I'm sure it's because of my age – I've been noticing a lot of women in my industry having babies and training safely the whole way through their pregnancies, and that has given me the confidence to think I could do the same thing too. One of my friends trained up until the day before she went into labour, and another girl I know went into early labour in the gym! I'm not saying that training throughout pregnancy is aspirational, or that I would necessarily want to do that, but it really gives me hope that you can still be just as active as long as you take precautions to keep your body safe. The fact that there are females who are pregnant and still squatting, lunging and walking the treadmill and doing it all safely really inspires me. It also means I would still be able to continue running our business through such a dramatic change to my body.

Of course, for any kind of public figure, sharing your journey to motherhood is always going to be stressful. It's exciting, but daunting at the same time, because it really is the unknown, and when people are watching you and scrutinising you doing anything you don't feel fully confident in, you're going to feel unnerved. Because there are a *lot* of opinions out there and people feel very happy to share them. There is no single, accepted textbook on how to raise a baby, so there are always going to be competing ideas on how to do it right. And on social media where people are so judgemental and critical anyway, I definitely feel like it will present a lot of challenges.

But I'm absolutely not shy about sharing the fact that I'm really looking forward to having a family and going on that journey with my audience. I feel like it will be such a privilege to be able to help support women going through such a huge change in their bodies, and I really hope that if I am lucky enough to get pregnant, I will be able to show others how you can keep active through pregnancy. I can't predict how it will affect me physically, but I feel like there is a really important story to be told there.

When and if we do decide to have kids, and if we are lucky enough to conceive, I'm going to be ready for it. As much as you can be of course. We were actually planning on starting trying in 2020, but we put everything back because of Covid. But it's definitely on the cards for us.

So, I guess my issue really isn't that it's what people expect of me, but more about how we all pile our own ideas of how people should live their lives on to each other. I do think it's something that's not talked about enough, and something which people can't seem to see is inappropriate to comment on. From a mental health perspective, none of us has any idea what someone else is going through, so sharing your ideas on what you think they should be doing is a really difficult thing for people to deal with.

I can identify with this from another period in my life, too. Growing up, I felt a lot of pressure around body image. As I talked about earlier in the book, I was known for being totally flat-chested while I was at school, and the boys always used to take the mickey out of me for it. It wasn't bullying or anything extreme – we probably all have some little thing that we were teased about when we were younger that has stuck with us in later life. I think the weight of expectation was that I would finally develop at some point and look a certain way. When I was young, the whole 'lad' culture was happening, with magazines like *Nuts* and *Zoo*, as well as the *Sun's* page 3. No one ever talked about bums back then, it was all boobs. So I did feel pressure around my body shape, and I can't tell you how much I just wanted a pair of boobs.

Even when I gained more confidence in my body in the gym, that pressure continued to niggle at me, and after a lot of thought and consideration, I ended up getting a boob job at the end of 2017. That was four years ago now, and sometimes looking back, I do think that perhaps some of the reasons behind my decision weren't quite what I'd feel

197

now and there are times when I think maybe I could have them out, even though I do love them. At the time, my biggest reason for doing it was because I felt so unconfident wearing certain clothes when I couldn't wear a bra. There was definitely a bit of a disconnect going on, because when I looked at other girls who had small boobs like mine, I'd think they looked amazing. But when it came to my own body, I just couldn't see myself like that, and all I could focus on was that I didn't like about my chest. In the gym, you can build muscle pretty much everywhere. You can get a bigger bum, legs and biceps, and I built curves on my bottom half that I didn't have before, but you can't train your boobs. I felt like I was completely disproportionate, that my body looked unbalanced, and that really affected the way I dressed and how uncomfortable I was with my body.

There is definitely a conflict. It was a choice I made entirely for myself and it definitely gave me confidence; I feel empowered by having made that decision and loving the results. But sometimes I do wonder if it was the right thing to do, because I should love my body just as it is. That is what I absolutely believe in, and sometimes, when I'm saying that to the world, I do think, well, is it a bit insincere because I've got these done? How do you square having a boob job with what I do truly believe about self-acceptance? It is a really tricky issue, and I go round and round in circles in my head about it. Ultimately, it made me happy, and I suppose at the end of the day, that is the only real thing that matters.

I was very transparent about my decision with my audience – I felt that was really important, so I vlogged and posted the whole experience of having a breast enlargement. That again was a funny one – I didn't want to hide it or lie, but equally I didn't want to be seen to be encouraging anyone else to do the same as it's such a personal decision. When I was looking into the procedure, there wasn't that much information out there that I felt I could trust, but I did come across one girl who had vlogged the process and I found it *so* helpful. I was like, wow, maybe I could also give others an insight into what is going to happen to them as it's so scary when it's such a complete unknown.

I think it's also important to say that I'm not ashamed of getting breast implants. I mean, the reality is that I could probably not have mentioned them and no one would have noticed. Before I had my boob job, I would wear two padded bras under a sports bra to make it look like I had something – anything – there. I felt I needed to do that just to make myself feel comfortable enough to leave the house. No one ever realised that I had absolutely no boobs. So all that happened was that I replaced the pads in my bra with implants in my boobs – from the outside I looked the same.

I don't like super-revealing clothes, and I certainly didn't get my boobs done so I could flash them around (not that there is anything wrong with that, it just wasn't my motivation). I would personally feel really uncomfortable if they did draw that kind of attention. There are so many times when I'll say to Romane, can you see anything in this sports bra, does it look inappropriate? You know, I'm going into a gym every day with a lot of guys, I don't want to have my flipping knockers out all the time, because it's sadly just going to draw one kind of attention and I'd prefer to be able to go about my day without guys looking at me that way. I just wanted to feel comfortable in myself and that my top half matched my bottom half.

Romane was very ambivalent about the whole thing and told me he didn't care either way. He always told me I was beautiful how I was, but that he would support any decision that I made about my own body. So he was supportive rather than encouraging. And thank God, because if he'd been really into the idea, I think I'd have been a bit like, you're not happy with me now then? He couldn't win really! But as usual he was amazing and there for me through the whole thing, holding my hand after the surgery and coming with me to the nurse for all the checks afterwards.

I would never say anything negative about anyone who wants to have any kind of cosmetic treatment that makes them feel good. Because if it makes them feel good that's bloody brilliant. End of. But it would also be so amazing if we could all find 100 per cent confidence in our unique beauty, so we didn't feel we needed that. I wasn't there in 2017 and I'm not sure I'm even there now – I'm definitely striving towards that as a goal and I really do believe in it. Like so many things to do with our looks, it's not straight-forward, but I also felt so much love from my community throughout the experience, and so many women were so kind to share their own cosmetic journeys with me, that it really made me realise that so many of us are in the same boat.

Another way that other people's expectations have affected me was the way in which so many people wrote me off as a young woman. Dealing with very low expectations can be just as difficult to cope with as feeling the weight of very high expectations. Because no one believed in me and they often told me that I would amount to nothing, I had zero confidence growing up. And it started so young. When I was five, my dad told me to put my hand up in class if I thought I knew the answer. But there was a maths teacher who then said that because I was wrong every time, I shouldn't keep putting my hand up, because it was clear I didn't know what I was talking about. My God, that has stayed with me. It's even with me a bit today. I still have this feeling that I shouldn't put my hand up because I'm inevitably going to be wrong, because I'm always wrong, and getting it wrong is really bad. And when I didn't get good grades and was always in the lowest sets, it felt as though those low expectations were being consistently met. After school, I had my hairdressing job where the boss made me feel like the smallest person on the planet, then I went into another job where that boss said that I'd never earn more than £16k. So during my younger years I definitely internalised the low expectations that other people pro-jected on to me, and that had a major impact on what I thought of myself. It wasn't a great start.

Why people dismiss you at such a young age is beyond me. The people I met had no idea what I was capable of and yet they thought they knew everything about my story and my future. It's crazy. What you can achieve and what you can do with your life is up to you, and you should never let anyone make you feel like a loser before you even start your journey. When I look back at stuff like that it's really strange. I mean it was adults, people who were my mum and dad's age, who said these things to me and made me feel that way, while I was just a young teenager who didn't have much confidence as it was. I just think it's odd – but I suppose it says more about them than me and they're probably unhappy, even now.

My expectations of what I could do and could achieve didn't really begin to shift until I spent a year on my own after so many years of being in relationships. I cannot tell you how important it is to spend time getting to know yourself and finding your inner voice in order to build up your own ideas of how you want to live your life beyond other people's expectations of you. If you're in a relationship that isn't taking you on the path you want for yourself, get out. Find yourself. It's the most amazing feeling. That was the first year that I had ever really been on my own, because I was in back-to-back relationships from the age of fifteen until my mid-twenties, and I was someone who would just go with the flow of what my partner wanted. After that year of being single, it was as if when it came to what I wanted out of life, no one could touch me. If anyone said anything bad about my choices, it just rolled off me, because I was so sure of who I was and so much clearer about what I wanted out of life.

Working on social media, I can see that there is a lot of pressure to achieve certain things by a certain age. That pressure is so difficult for young people, and I am so happy that social media wasn't around in my younger years, as it allowed me the time to get to know myself, make mistakes, grow and develop without the comparison culture. Social media today can sometimes make young people expect instant success, and some kids are leaving school and uni thinking that they're going to be earning a lot of money and getting promotions immediately. The problem with that is that if they don't achieve success in their twenties, they think they've failed and their life is over. But look at us! I didn't even set up my Instagram account until I was twenty-six. I'd had two other careers and already lost a fiancé by then! My success didn't even start building until my late twenties and I'm only hitting my stride now in my thirties.

Both Romane and I would say that we didn't mature until our late twenties. Romane always says that he was a boy until he met me, and it took him a long time to grow up and stop doing boy things and messing around. Similarly, I had no concern about my thirties and forties when I was young. I know that other people do mature earlier and you do see very young people in fitness who have already built businesses by their early twenties and are already focused on their long-term success. But what I would say is that it's not a race. You can always turn things around, start new ventures and find your focus, regardless of your age. We have to lose this idea that success comes quickly for everyone; it's much more of a journey, so if you hit thirty and you're not there yet, don't lose faith.

As a really good example, Romane and I were looking at a couple on social media this week. The account was started about a year ago by a guy in his late forties and he's already got a million followers. He's got a great physique and posts workouts, same as me, sometimes with his wife who is also in her forties. They have lots of kids, some of whom are grown up now. Back in the day, no one would have thought that a couple in their late forties could reinvent themselves and find such great success in fitness later in life, but today the opportunities don't end at a certain age. Ten years ago, the internet and social media were a young person's thing, but that is just not the case anymore and it's so cool to see people from every generation blossoming and building success – it's never too late.

Things happen in their own time, and I think a lot of anxiety is created by trying to push for something when it doesn't seem to be happening 'on schedule'. Romane and I would never have been successful in the same way when we were younger. Romane was a proper lad in his early twenties! He'd have been off doing this, that and the other and he wouldn't have appreciated me or been ready to focus on building a business. And I needed my year of being single to really work out what I wanted out of life. We needed to meet each other and work as a team to get to where we are now; coming together and sharing a passion has enabled us to build our success. So it happened at the right time, no earlier and no later.

When it comes to my expectations for the future, I feel like the sky's the limit. When I look back on what we have managed to achieve over the past six years, I now believe we can do anything. Last year we decided to make a massive change and move to Dubai, which certainly wasn't something I had seen coming. But life takes you on unusual routes, so I've started to realise there's not that much point in making long-term plans. Instead you just have to be open to opportunities as and when they come. Back when I was younger, I thought that was it for me – a life in an unfulfilling job with a partner who didn't value me. I had no idea what I could achieve if I really put my mind to it, so now I wouldn't even try to guess where we're going to be in ten years. Anything is possible. I have no expectations, other than that it's going to be a lot of hard work, with lots of excitement and wonderful experiences ahead, and Romane and I will take it all step by step and hand in hand.

STEP SIX RECAP:

- The expectations we have for our lives can cast a long shadow over our happiness. When you feel like you're slipping behind or having a worse quality of life than other people, it can make you feel like a failure, even when you're doing really well. Comparing what you have – the size of your house or the type of holiday you can afford – to what other people have is really easy but not really relevant. We are all on different journeys and all start from different places, so you just can't compare.

- It's often other people's expectations that create pressure. Even though the world has changed so much, there are still a lot of traditional views out there when it comes to things like marriage and kids. Other people's assumptions of what you will and won't do shouldn't have an impact on your decision-making.

- Getting to know yourself is such an important part of development and can help you to identify what it is you really want. Often, if you're not the most outspoken person, you can end up going with the flow in a relationship and not asserting yourself. Having time to yourself should be seen as a precious thing – there is so much emphasis on dating and finding 'the one', but when you're young I think focusing on yourself should be your priority.

- With body image, the expectations of what we should look like come from all angles. From our peers at school and college, from magazines and social media, from TV and films. It's hard to escape, and even harder when you've internalised those expectations. Ultimately, every woman should feel empowered to do whatever makes them feel amazing.

- There is no age limit for success. In this day and age, when TikTok stars are becoming millionaires in their teens, it can sometimes feel that if you haven't made it by the time you are thirty, it's all over for you. That is just not the case. It's never too late and it's not a race to get to where you're going.
- Having low expectations of yourself can be just as toxic as the pressure of having high expectations. It felt like no one believed in me when I was younger, but they were wrong. Ignore everyone else and go about your journey to success. There are always going to be people who make you feel small, but anyone can improve their life if they're prepared to work hard at something they are passionate about.

STEP SIX TO PHYSICAL STRENGTH: THE LOW-DOWN ON INJURIES

*How to avoid them, how to heal them and how to
keep your mojo going throughout*

Romane

Of all the different factors that can damage your mojo and
undermine your consistency, injury has the greatest potential to derail your fitness goals. Because if you hurt yourself,
there is nothing you can do but let it run its course. Obviously there are steps you can take to help yourself through
recovery, from physio to sports massage, but injuries,
whether they are chronic or training-related, need to be
rested and taken seriously. The most obvious (yet not mentioned enough) way to deal with injury is to not get one in
the first place! I have had some serious gym-related injuries

along the way, including one that led to a six-week stay in hospital, and I have definitely been guilty in the past of not heeding my own advice. But as I've matured and gained experience, there are now certain precautions I take which are set in stone.

Firstly, the absolute golden rule is to train within your means and progress slowly. Your job is to build up to your goals, not sprint to them, however impatient you might feel. Man, I've been there. But the way Lisa and I train now is consistent but gradual. In fact, Lisa has always done that as she is naturally cautious; in her six years of lifting she has never had one serious or even medium-level training-related injury. If that doesn't tell you everything you need to know, I don't know what will. Lisa's injury-free experience is a testament to taking your time. She will never lift a weight that is too heavy for her and will always come at a set from a lower weight and add if she feels she is able to.

She is also really, really focused on her technique. Form is everything when you are trying to ensure your training remains injury-free. That means ensuring that your form is perfect before increasing your weight in any context, either with free weights or on a machine. When I talk about form, what I mean is where you put your feet when you lift, the angles of your joints and the muscles that you engage to make a movement. On the machines it's how

211

you do a rep (generally engaging many more muscles than just the targeted area) and your posture. It is vital that you take the time to learn what you are doing to your body during exercise and how to perfectly position yourself to ensure you're protected while building muscle. I think if everyone took the time to properly look into what they were doing, we would reduce injuries by a huge proportion. You can learn all of this by yourself, through YouTube and beyond, but you can also ask a PT to help you for a few sessions for some hands-on adjustments to make sure you are getting the foundations of your weight training journey bang on. Aside from more debilitating training-related injuries, I think many of the niggles that people tend to get from gym work are down to very small elements being just that bit off – a slight angle here, a few centimetres marginally off of your foot placement there. But when you are lifting heavy weights, those tiny differences can cause all sorts of problems.

I can't emphasise enough how important it is to not have an ego in the gym. I started lifting at thirteen, and along the way I've done every stupid thing you could possibly imagine trying to impress my bros and myself. Lifting weights that are beyond your ability isn't impressive to anyone, because you will ruin yourself, and three weeks on the sofa is going to absolutely trash all of your progress. I've been lifting for twenty years and I can absolutely say that humility is one of the biggest gifts I've been given over that time.

Another piece of advice to anyone starting training is to respect the rest days. Post-workout muscle recovery is so incredibly fundamental to staying injury-free. Your muscles are working all the time to repair the little tears that resistance exercise makes to the myofibrils, but when you overtrain you compound all of those tiny tears into an injury. Most muscle strains happen because the muscle has either been stretched beyond its limit or has been forced to contract too strongly. In mild cases only a few fibres are stretched or torn and the muscle itself stays intact and is able to perform normal functions – you'll feel a bit sore, but it will heal in due course. In more serious cases, too many fibres are stretched, as well as blood vessels, filling the area with blood, and that is when you are going to have to sit out your sessions.

When that happens, the muscle's first response is to seal off the area of damage, ensuring repair is focused at the sight of the injury. During the initial phase, you will find that inflammation sets in and you will feel swelling, pain and potentially a sensation of heat as the body's natural response to soft tissue damage kicks in. The inflammation reduces tissue infection, so you should see it as part of the healing process. During this stage, complete rest (no stretching)

213

can help reduce pain and control the bleeding and swelling: think RICE (rest, ice, compression and elevation). You should also consult a specialist as soon as you can to put together a tailored programme of rehab.

The next stage is known as the destruction phase, when white blood cells called macrophages are introduced to the area. In Greek, macrophage literally means 'large eater', and what these cells do is digest any dead cells caused by the injury. Next up, muscle steam cells flood the area and turn into myoblast cells, which fuse into tubes which will become the regenerated muscle fibres. In addition, new blood vessels and nerves are generated, which peaks around two weeks after your injury.

Around a month or two after the trauma, your muscle will be in the remodelling phase. This is when the fibres and connective tissues mature, and this stage is really important for how the scar tissue is organised. Typical muscle tissue is oriented in straight lines like logs, but regenerated scar tissue can be organised randomly as a mixture of connective tissue and muscle fibres, which can cause a clump-like shape that may limit movement and strength going forward. What can help to improve the organisation of the regenerated fibres is keeping active (not back to training the muscle, but keeping the body moving). While the muscle could still be sore and you might feel that you should rest, starting with low-level exercise is vital to improve the function of the new muscle tissue. When your body detects that a repaired structure is weaker than it should be, it automatically stimulates additional new tissue to strengthen and support the still-healing tissue until it can meet the pressures you put it under. So if you just put your feet up, waiting for it to heal, your body will think, 'job done!' and it won't work to further strengthen the muscle. But if you slowly start to move again, you will ensure an increased blood supply to the muscle, which will provide an optimum amount of oxygen and nutrients to the injury site and stimulate your body to continue to build new tissue. To then bring the muscle back up to its previous strength, or as close as possible, active rehab, or slow, progressive training is the name of the game. The key here is being able to differentiate between a low level of soreness and actual pain – you should never train with pain in any instance, especially not after an injury.

What I tell all of my clients is that every single serious injury I've ever had has happened on a day when I shouldn't have been in the gym – on days when I was yawning on the way to the gym, having come off the back of multiple days of training, when my body was so fatigued and my nervous system was frayed. For whatever reason, I'd convinced myself that I needed to go in that day, because I was preparing for an event or working towards another goal, and I let my own ego take over. 'I'll be fine, it's just one more session.' No. You won't be fine. If your body is telling you to rest, you have to listen to it. Every time I've ignored my body in that situation, something bad has happened.

As for my injuries, I've had a stage two pec tear which was quite rough. At stage three you have to have an operation to reattach the tendon, and my stage two was at the more severe end of the scale, so it was incredibly painful, bruised everywhere and really difficult to rebuild from. I could still continue my cardio and training my legs, as that didn't put any pressure on the muscle. I gave my arms a break for a few weeks, as they're attached to your shoulder which is attached to your chest muscle and I didn't want to stretch it at all initially, but after that, I just did what I could. One of the benefits of weightlifting is that you can target different areas of the body while resting other areas, meaning that when you are injured you can protect the area that is damaged while ramping it up elsewhere. I kept my nutrition the same because I was still training to a similar volume, but I really did protect my pec muscle and took a slow, measured approach to active rehab several weeks after the initial tear.

Another injury to my foot put me in a hospital bed for six weeks, and that was just a different level of rehab and there was no way I could train at all. I decided the only option was to go with it and not fight the situation. I wasn't able to keep up my nutrition in hospital, so I just ate whatever I wanted and I think that helped me psychologically. There was no point trying to eat six meals a day, so I just ate what my friends and family brought me, enjoyed it, and knew that when I healed, I could go 100% and get my physique back. There was a moment during that experience when I was told that I might not be able to compete again – and even that there was a chance of amputation – so it was absolutely imperative that I focused on getting myself healthy again rather than trying to rush back to fitness.

When you do make it back to the gym post-injury, it's back to the basics. That will strengthen the particular area that you have a weakness in. Rather than just hitting the gym, consult with a sports physio and take on board their advice. If there is one thing I would go back and do differently, it would be to do a lot more research into the mechanics of the body. While you might be desperate to get under the bar and start doing impressive-looking lifts, take a minute and remember that it's your bodyweight movements that provide you with the foundation for everything. They are what will make the most difference at the beginning as your body gets used to specific movements, muscles stretch and strengthen to allow specific movements and your brain fine-tunes the movement pathways. Just simply squatting down and touching your bum off a bench doesn't look very hardcore, but the truth is, that's what going to get you to the next step, that's your foundation. Instead of squatting under a bar (which let's be clear is 20kg without any weight on, and for a beginner that is pretty heavy), work on your squat form. If you've only been squatting to go to the loo thus far, you are going to find it hard and you are going to need to work on it. Most people are not ready for a squat bar; in all my years in the gym, I would say that the vast majority of people that I see squatting under the bar do so with terrible technique. *Build up to it, don't sprint to it.*

It's worth mentioning that there is a huge mental health aspect to injury. Anyone who trains in a way that supports their happiness and wellbeing will find that injury can really cause their mood to dip, and it's easy to slip into a mild depression. If you can continue to at least do something safely, I really believe you should. And while injuries require rest, it's so important to continue to get the blood flowing to a damaged muscle as that gives it the best chance of repair. As soon as you can start moving, even if it's just a walk around the block, you should. Always remember that your body adapts to the stimulus it is given, so if you sit at home for two months, feeling miserable, you will find that the muscle will weaken as you aren't asking it to do anything. Anytime the body can catabolise muscle tissue it will, and that of course is the opposite of strengthening a muscle. Keeping even a low level of movement going will also support your mental health as the feel-good hormones are released again.

Coming back from injury is all about taking your time and not competing with where you were before you hurt yourself. It sounds like a cliché, but you have to be kind to yourself. You have to let the injury run its course and allow your body to repair. What is worth highlighting is that every time I've had an injury, the lasting effects have been more psychological than physical. While I've always wanted to get back into the gym as soon as possible, you can't help but be affected by the trauma and you carry a heavy weight of apprehension, because you just don't want to be back there again. Even when I've healed physically, I've found there was a big psychological mountain to climb to get back to proper training, because you are so gun-shy about pushing yourself. I think the thing to remember is that your body and mind are connected, and that with any physical pain or damage that you sustain, there is also going to be a mental fallout. We need to try and support both sides of that con-nection when we are injured and not focus exclusively on the physical element.

STEP SEVEN TO MENTAL STRENGTH: NEVER TAKE YOUR MIND OR BODY FOR GRANTED

How we've trained ourselves in gratitude

In this final step we wanted to give a little insight into our life and the long-term reality of living strong. As a couple, we support each other every step of the way, and while we are so motivated to build our business and reach more and more people with our message, we are also learning to live in the present and focus on the smaller moments. In this final chapter we have come together to offer our advice to anyone who wants to change their life for the better and maintain those changes forever.

Lisa & Romane xx

Forever Strong

Lisa: While we go on (and on and on) about the power of short-term goals, there is obviously still a place for

222

dreaming big and reaching the top of the mountain. One of the flaws of most conventional diet and fitness books is that they devote too little time to discussing what happens at the finish line, or the 'after'. As I've mentioned before, everything I practise and preach is about achieving trans-formational changes to your entire lifestyle, so for me there is no 'after' in the sense that once you've reached your goal you can't just go back to how you were living before. If you want to continue reaping the rewards of the results, you have to remain on this journey forever. That doesn't mean a life of endless restrictions and deprivation; it's about find-ing your ideal personal balance and what works for you. But you do have to have your eyes open to what your life is going to look like if you stick with your goals.

To maintain the muscle you have built, to feel strong, healthy and energetic, and to continue to feel the huge mood and confidence boost that exercise gives you, you're going to have to eat well, sleep well, hydrate and continue to be consistent in your fitness plan. Muscle mass declines very quickly. Even fitness professionals and athletes who train 300 days a year will start to lose muscle strength within three weeks if they stop working out. It's just not a dip-in-and-out thing. Of course you can have breaks and come back to exercise, but it may feel like you're back on the ground floor again, which can sometimes feel demoralising.

223

Living strong is a holistic choice, which impacts every area of your life, so I don't want to give you false expectations. If you follow my plan at the end of the book, that is just the start, to get you into the right mindset for your new lifestyle, so it's definitely worth thinking about what comes next and whether you are ready to jump in.

The diet side of the coin is something that gets a lot of attention in the context of maintenance, because for a lot of people making good choices with food the majority of the time is something that is challenging due to the myriad emotional issues that come with eating (and drinking).

Romane: I have a history of emotional overeating and I do struggle to stay disciplined without a goal, so I really empathise with those who find their diet an issue. One of the key elements of success in this case is to be able to find joy in something other than food, because the thing is, food never lets you down. That first biscuit is always going to taste nice and put a smile on your face, no matter what else is going on around you. In order to be successful in the long term, you can't rely on only food to do that for you. But if you can find something you really enjoy, you will in turn find the strength to remove your emotions from the choices you make around your nutrition.

Lisa: I absolutely understand why so many people have become anti-diet. At the minute, more and more people are creating awareness about the flaws in fad diets, whereas back in the day, social media wasn't around to critique all the terrible food trends and dangerous diet books. So the whole conversation is definitely changing. I do agree that the faddy, insanely extreme diets of the past need to *stay* in the past. But that doesn't mean that everything you see on social media should be trusted either – there is a lot of dodgy advice online, pure and simple.

It's really important for me to be honest here and say that what you eat still has a big impact on your results. It would be disingenuous for me to tell you to expect changes without making changes to your diet. There's a bit of a movement right now on social media which basically suggests you can eat what you want and still be whatever you want. People are literally trying to have their cake and eat it, and I don't believe that's good advice. There has to be a middle way and you have to be realistic – you're not going to achieve X without doing Y, it's just simple chemistry. If there's not enough protein in your diet, if you're carrying a higher percentage of body fat because you're consuming a higher number of calories and you're not ensuring a good balance of essential vitamins and minerals in your diet, then you aren't going to build muscle or be able to see it visibly at an optimum level.

When people say that diets don't work, it's often because the diet they are talking about is overly restrictive and only runs for a short time. A lot of people think, 'I'll go on a diet for six weeks,' and they are ultra-strict during that time, or for as long as they can manage. They will remove all the things they really love and feel miserable about it. They then inevitably fall back into their old ways. But if you look at your nutrition as a long-term deal, you just don't need to do that. The slower approach is to find a new balance where you can enjoy the things you like in moderation, so you don't start obsessing about what you're missing out on and so don't fall off the wagon. If you have a sweet tooth, a reasonable portion of dark chocolate from time to time isn't going to have an impact on your overall results. If you really like a drink, a glass of red wine with your dinner here and there won't totally derail your efforts. Obviously, you won't lose body fat as quickly as going on a diet which basically starves you (it's worth noting that crash diets also deplete muscle mass, especially if you don't eat enough protein). But the changes you make over a longer period of time with your new, more balanced lifestyle will be so much more sustainable and long-lasting.

The whole idea of 'going on a diet' is just a waste of time. It has to be more along the lines of, 'I'm permanently changing the way I eat while still incorporating the things I love without going wild.' Not quite as catchy, right? But that is the only thing that's going to work, because it's not workable (or in any way desirable, who would want to live like that?!) to deprive yourself for weeks and months. More often than not, that kind of restriction also leads to a bad relationship with food. You may find that food and eating begins to control you, everything becomes quite pressurised and a lot of anxiety around your diet can build up, because it is really excruciating to continually deny yourself the things you love. Cycles of being 'good' and being 'bad', going from restriction to binges, can lead to a host of negative feelings about yourself, and that goes against the entire reason that you started on this journey in the first place. It was meant to be about feeling stronger and better, wasn't it? Changes to your diet don't have to be all or nothing, and over the years you can find that sweet spot where you can indulge and it doesn't undermine your progress because you have set up such a solid, healthy structure to your lifestyle. The thing is, that takes more than six weeks, I'm sorry to say.

Romane: There are always compromises to make if you want to achieve things in the gym. That is just fact. It also goes for making improvements to your lifts and increasing your stamina and energy levels, not just the way you look. As a couple, we have found a balance by always having one midweek day and one weekend day where we aren't as strict with what we eat. Unless either of us are in prep for a particular goal, on Wednesdays and Saturdays we will always have something that we love.

Lisa: I find it pretty easy to stick to that, because I always know that if I fancy something specific, I can always have it soon. Not in ten weeks' time. Knowing that I can eat what I want at some point in the week also kind of takes the craving out of it. Of course, every now and again we will go out a few nights in a row or get takeaways. And we know that the next day we might not feel our absolute best, but you have to remember that you don't have to make the perfect choices every single day of your life. We will have something on a Wednesday and something at the weekend, and we like to do it that way because when we eat junk food, we absolutely *feel* the impact of it the next day. We have 100 per cent reached the point where a treat or two makes no difference to how we look, but if we eat food that is nutritionally poorer, it will take it out of us for a day or two after. It will mean that we struggle to get up and out in the morning, that we will have training sessions where we're not progressing, and not pushing ourselves to our full potential, and that we're not enjoying our work as much because we're so sluggish and tired. It can come as a bit of a shock when you're so used to eating a diet that doesn't nourish you that certain foods can make you feel that way. For so many people it has become the norm to feel 'cloudy' all day long and lack motivation.

Romane: Most people walk around dehydrated, under-nourished, exhausted after not enough good sleep, hitting up caffeine to keep them going through the day. But it is not normal to feel shit all the time.

Lisa: That's why I get so frustrated when people say to me, 'I couldn't live like you do, I couldn't eat like that all the time.' I wish they only knew how good they could feel if they did, and anyway, I do still have what I want. The truth is, while I enjoy junk from time to time, I so prefer the way I feel when I eat nutrient-dense food that I just don't want it that much. If you have never known what it feels like to be clear-headed and fresh *all the time*, it's hard to imagine how incredibly different your life could be, how much more energy you could have and how much better you would feel in yourself. If people knew that, it would help them stick to making good choices in the long term.

Romane: Lisa and I thrive on routine and structure, and that applies to our nutrition too, as it enables us to be more productive with our lives. When we know what we're having for lunch and dinner, we never get hangry. When you don't have the right food and you're caught out, it's impossible to be productive and positive and it's hard to have an uplifting mood. We like to get our nutrition in and know it's sorted. Even if we're going out for breakfast or dinner, having a structure means everything else just falls into place.

Ditch the Haters; a Support Network Matters

Romane: I personally think that it doesn't really matter if your partner shares the same nutritional or fitness goals as you. What is hard is when they don't offer you support or encouragement. And that goes for anyone in your life that you are close to. From my own experience, the minute you decide to do something positive for yourself, you may find that those around you try and knock you off course. They ask, 'Why would you want to do that anyway?' The problem with changing is that often the people around you stay the same, and watching you make your incredible progress can make them feel negative about their own reality – and this may make them want to pull you down.

When I was PT'ing, the number one reason why people who had done amazingly well fell off their diet plan was because people close to them tried to push them back into their old lifestyle. They would make them feel so guilty that in the end, they would cave. It would be sisters, husbands, generally anyone who wasn't able to do it themselves. It's not nice to think about, but from my experience, the people closest to you can be the biggest challenge to keeping on track in the long term.

Lisa: One of Romane's clients gained muscle so naturally, she was just genetically programmed to do it – she had something really special. But as she started building her strength, her friends began to constantly put her down for her progress; they couldn't work out why she was making compromises to achieve something which they didn't deem desirable. In the end, she stopped training completely for a long while. We see it so much in our Facebook group. People post saying, my mum said this or my best friend said that and it knocked my confidence. But here's the thing: other people's opinions on how you look are nothing to do with how you choose to live. If weightlifting and building a strong body make you feel and look great, that is all anyone else needs to know.

Romane: As soon as I started competing, I became pretty strict with my diet and I really enjoyed that challenge and doing something for myself. The first thing I noticed was how mean everyone around me suddenly became about it. I couldn't work out why they were trying to pull me down, because what is it to them if I don't eat a sausage roll for my dinner? It's up to me what I do and how I live my life. However bad it was for me, I do think that kind of response is even worse for girls.

Lisa: It happens to me all the time. I'll go to a party or a lunch and I'll be asked, 'Ooo, can you have that?' or 'Are you allowed to eat this?' Then it will be, 'Go on, try it,' or 'You look like you could do with a bit of cake.' My response is always the same: of course I could have it if I wanted it, it's not like I have the police coming round if I have a slice of cake! But for me, if it's a choice between that cake and achieving something that I really, *really* want, I'm going to leave it. Thanks, though.

Romane: Part of living strong is that you're going to have to put up with people trying to make you eat an extra piece of cake for the rest of your life. You start looking and feeling better and more often than you would believe, the response from others is to try and get you to quit your plan.

Lisa: I think understanding the psychology behind why people are trying to knock you off your track is important for helping you to resist the pressure.

Romane: From my perspective, when I try to stick to a diet, or we do it together, I know how much potential we have inside of us. Potential to build our business and inspire other people, potential to create great, engaging content and potential to develop our bodies to feel and look amazing. That's what I'm always thinking about. I know that if we make those compromises, something really special will come from it.

Setbacks and Pauses

Romane: No one is perfect and we both know what it's like to fall off the wagon. Last year I lost a lot of motivation and fell off hard. Only for about two or three months, which in the grand scheme of things isn't that much, but the change in my body was pretty major. I literally looked like a different person. Being locked down and not having access to the gym affected me in ways I didn't think were possible, and I spent the whole summer feeling sorry for myself and overindulging every day. Competing can definitely have an impact on your mentality and lead you to believe that if you're not 'stage lean' then you're fat, and, conversely, if you're not adding muscle each year, you're too skinny. After years of keeping my discipline together it was really hard to come to terms with not being able to maintain my lifestyle goals. But I managed to get back on the horse and am working really hard to stay in this lane for now. I'm saying all of this just to reassure anyone else who has achieved some of their goals and changed their lifestyle only to slip back at some point. You can always get back to where you felt amazing – just start setting those short-terms goals again.

Lisa: In an ideal world you would build a structure and routine which is manageable and sustainable, so when you do decide to enjoy yourself, it doesn't even register as a blip. After we've had a pause in our usual routine, we will always make sure that we train, drink a lot of water, sleep and try to get back to our structure sooner rather than later. Not because we feel guilty or pressured into it because of our jobs, but because it makes us feel better. Even on holiday, we still keep an element of discipline. We always get up early and go for a morning walk, which we absolutely love, and we'll do some kind of cardio during the day, either in or out of the gym. As we're active people, that's what we like to do, because it makes us feel fresh and energetic. It's definitely not like, 'Oh no, we've eaten too much pizza, we need to work out.' It's because we like the feeling it gives us. We never feel guilty about anything on holiday, but keeping just a bit of discipline going allows us to slip easily back into our usual routine.

Romane: Sometimes you have to let down your hair, otherwise what's the point in living? You've got to enjoy those special moments. If you can't have an ice-cold beer at the beach what's the point?! That's what you work for after all. But that doesn't mean we can't be active as well. Generally, when you speak to someone who doesn't go to the gym, or who is overweight, they might say to you something like, 'I've got to lose weight, but I can't run,' as if running is the only thing anyone can do to lose weight. But we never run! We only ever walk. And we've both got down to 5 per cent body fat just from walking.

Lisa: People don't see walking outside or on a treadmill as being a way to reduce body fat, but it's the best form of exercise. You don't have to 'go for walks' to incorporate more walking into your life. Always take the stairs and don't catch the bus – just walk at any opportunity and, over time, it will make a huge impact. It doesn't sound that exciting, does it, but I never find it boring. I feel the same about the gym – however many leg presses and bicep curls I do, I still get that buzz.

Romane: For me, the gym is the best part of the day, and everything else kind of revolves around it. It makes you feel so good. You just know that when you walk out of the gym, you're going to feel on top of the world, endorphins pumping, feeling that amazing sense of achievement.

Lisa: I never get bored of that. But I do understand that for some people, the constant repetition of the same exercises can start to feel monotonous and that keeping to the same routine can become dull after a while. That's why we mix up our gym routines and jumble everything. That's what keeps it interesting. We're always adding new techniques and changing the splits. We might do a stint on specific muscle groups, but then we might change it to a push-pull-legs (a simple training method in which the body is split into three parts: the push is the upper body pushing muscles, the pull the upper body pulling muscles. Every training session is split to focus on one of these three muscle groups) to keep your body guessing. You can't hit that plateau when you're always changing things, so for us it's never a standard 'three sets of ten' – we're always throwing new things in there. I never want to just coast. To this day, I train more because of the way it makes me feel, but I also like to add more weight in a session. Some sessions I won't be able to go past a certain weight, while other sessions I will. But I do like to try to push myself in terms of strength to keep me motivated. I don't have a number in my mind in terms of weight that I can lift that I'm heading towards, but I definitely am always striving to reach new goals. Even when you're in maintenance, you can keep challenging yourself just that bit further every week, every month, every year.

Romane: That's definitely true, but you do have to take into account the weightlifter's cycle and accept that the initial progress you make will slow down, often almost to a stop. The reality is that you can't just keep pushing one area of the body in a linear upwards trajectory. You might be doing a squat say for twelve weeks, and then you'll reach a peak and perhaps your knees can't take any more. So you start doing a leg press until you reach your peak there, and then you might move on to lunges and six months later you might find yourself back at squats again. You are always improving in some area.

Lisa: With my exercises, I get to a certain weight and I can never get past that. But like Romane says, you improve at something else, then you go back to where you started, so there is always progress to be found. With weightlifting, it's not like you ever finish, there's always something to work on.

Romane: That's also the reason why it can be difficult to gauge long-term progress in the gym. Women can expect to gain about three or four pounds of muscle tissue in their first year of building, double that for men. Then after that it's a pound a year or even less. And that's only if you're consistent, go 300 days a year, eat all your meals and do all your lifts. So while you're putting in all this work, you may only gain a relatively small amount of muscle mass when you get into a long-term relationship with the gym. Let's say you're doing the bench press. You might be hitting ten reps on the same weight for four months. Then after four months, you might be able to put on a tiny weight each side, and that will add to your body overall.

It's much harder for women to gain muscle no matter what their age, and for men in their mid- to late thirties, progress starts to fall off and then dramatically decline as their testosterone level drops. But you *can* still make progress. You can improve your form, you can improve your stamina and of course you can always improve your overall fitness. Just ask triathletes who reach peak fitness, then two weeks after the race they're almost back to square one and have to start all over again. They might do the same time for ten years before making any improvement. Now that requires some patience.

Lisa: There is definitely a confidence side to progress, which I have struggled with over the years. I can sometimes be a little negative about my abilities, and I tell myself I can't do things from time to time. I go through waves. Some days I get to the gym and feel like I can do anything – chuck another weight on, I'm on a roll! – then sometimes when I'm having a bit of a wobble, I'll be like, no, no, I don't think I can do that. And Romane will be like, c'mon, you can do it. I'd say I'm generally more up than down, but sometimes I just get those little negative Nancies that can stand in the way of your potential.

Romane: That's improved over the years, because when I first met Lisa she was still new to training and there wasn't much self-belief in anything. I'd be like, let's go up to the next set and put some more weight on, and she would always be saying, no, no, I can't do that. But now, more often than not, she'll have a go. Unless she gives me *the look* and I know I better put the weight back down! But I know she can do it, I have confidence in her.

Lisa: Training with someone who can be that cheerleader for you, whether it's a friend, partner or PT, is really amazing for helping to push you to the next stage and combat any lack of self-belief. While I also enjoy training on my own, it's never quite as fun as when we train together.

I think it's also really important to talk about the mental strength side of maintenance, because that is a muscle that you just can't take for granted or feel like you're 'finished' dealing with. Even though I've come so far with my self-confidence, I still have my ups and downs, both in the gym and in terms of our business. I definitely had a crisis of confidence last year, which kind of took me by surprise as I felt I'd moved forward from that place. I think it was because everything had been sailing along before lockdown and I was feeling safe in my comfort zone, even though we were building and taking new steps. We had launched the app, it was going well and I felt confident in all aspects of what we were offering. Then the pandemic came, and everything did a complete one-eighty. As home workouts became the lifeline for everyone, I was thrown into an area that I didn't have much experience in and didn't really know how to approach.

I had never done classes before, and I felt there was an immense pressure on me, and that definitely knocked my confidence big time. I found myself stuck into a real cycle of comparison, watching other fitness professionals and influencers excel. There are so many people who are amazing at bringing the kind of energy you need to keep everyone's motivation high and a class flowing. As a personality, I'm just not 'out there' or loud or good at revving up a room, and I'm also just not a fake it 'til you make it kind of person. If I can't do it, I can't do it. I'm not going to lie. Some people have that amazing energy for classes and I didn't feel like I had that. It was like, God, I'm not good enough for this. Why do people even follow me when I can't even do this? It really hit me bad. It's so worth remembering that even though you feel better about yourself and have climbed that mountain in terms of your self-confidence and mental health, just like in the gym, you can backslide. There is absolutely nothing wrong with that – in fact, I think it is inevitable. Having a lack of self-belief and your brain always reverting to a place of insecurity and negative self-talk is a habit, and habits are hard to break but very easy to take up again. I had to pick myself up from that and it took me a bit of time because it bashed me a little bit. Now I'm back in my groove at the gym, I feel much better. But although it was a baptism of fire, I do now have a new string to my bow, and if we ever have a lockdown again, I would feel much more confident about taking at-home classes, because I know that I can do it. You have to take the positives – I would never have done that if it hadn't been for the pandemic, so there is no point dwelling on the fact I lost my footing a bit with my confidence.

Grateful for the Little Moments

Lisa: I think one of the things that has really helped me navigate my mental health and leave many of the bad habits behind has been to really focus on living in the present. The past is the past, the future hasn't happened yet, so take a breath and look around you today. Having goals is a great thing, and stretching towards a different future for yourself if you're not satisfied with your life is something I would always recommend. But I've definitely been lost in that treadmill to tomorrow, especially at the start of our business when it felt like every day all we were doing was chasing, chasing, working, working towards the dream. During those years we rarely took time out to be in the present, away from anything that wasn't driving towards the future. But since lockdown in particular, our mindset has changed.

Romane and I had all these plans for the next step for our business and life, and they didn't pan out because of lockdown. Instead of letting that feel like a massive setback, we decided to sell our family home and take a leap, moving abroad for new opportunities in a pivot that came out of nowhere. I know what you're thinking: the medium was right! Spooky, isn't it? For now, we are really happy, but who knows what will happen as the months pass, and of course I miss my family. But I learned that there is no point

241

in being so obsessed with the shape of a future which for whatever reason might not even happen. Now we have taken that breather and made the effort to stop and smell the roses, we focus much more on how grateful we are for everything that we have and that has happened. Yes, we have worked damn hard for it, but we don't take a single thing for granted. When you are so driven towards a single goal, sometimes if feels like the blinkers are on and it's really easy to forget to celebrate the amazing moments that happen along the way.

Romane: I know this is going to sound cheesy, but the number one thing I'm grateful for is Lisa. Appreciating each other and being constantly aware of how lucky you are to have important people in your life is really the first step towards gratitude.

Lisa: Working, living and training with your partner can be intense – while most couples have only spent so much time together over the past couple of years, we have been in each other's pockets basically since we met each other. It is so important to take time for each other – I think that's one of the secrets – even if it's just twenty seconds for a kiss and a cuddle. It's tough when you have a business like ours on social media, because it's all go go go, and you've got your phone in your hand all day long. The day can just run away with you and you might find you haven't said a word to each other for hours, even though you have been in the same room. So we definitely try to be more present for each other.

Romane: The first time I met Lisa, I said to her, 'you're going to be the biggest fitness influencer in the UK'. I have always seen a life like this for us and have always believed in Lisa.

Lisa: Romane has always had that vision – it's one of the things I found so attractive about him when I met him. For me, though, I still can't believe how far I've come. In my business, in my life, what I've achieved. It's just amazing. It can even be hard to remember where we are now, because I don't see myself in the same way that other people see me. Some mornings I wake up and I can't believe it. How did we do it? It's crazy. We started this whole thing six years ago, but I just didn't have the imagination to see us here. Not that I didn't believe in us, it's just that I didn't know it was possible, because of where I've come from. When you start investing in your mental and physical strength, you will see a potential you literally couldn't have dreamed of. I had no idea what I was capable of and it still astonishes me to this day.

If I can do it, so can you. I really hope that our story inspires you to think about your mindset and all the different ways you might be limiting yourself and your life. Of course, just as there isn't one ideal body type, there isn't one ideal version of mental strength, and your journey and potential will be completely unique to you. But you can absolutely go beyond what you might have once thought was the best you could ever achieve. As a final thought, I want to say that just as the way you look doesn't define you, neither does what you do for a living or how much you have or any of the outward showing trappings of life. Happiness and fulfilment are personal and intimate feelings and not things that anyone else can gauge.

My journey is my journey – it's not anyone else's and it won't resonate with everyone. I started out super-slim, massively insecure and pretty lost in terms of where my life was going. My progress has been to gain lean muscle, something which has been really tough for my body type, build my confidence and become an entrepreneur. I try to motivate other people with my story and show how much of a process it all is. You have to be patient and consistent, with both your physical and mental strength, as neither are going to change overnight. There is no magic pill, it's just hard work, compromise and staying focused on the short-term goals. It's taken me six years to gain 10kg of muscle and to start to leave some of the worst of my mental struggles behind. Every step has built on the one before to get me to where I am now: strong both inside and out.

STEP SEVEN RECAP:

- If you want to continue to reap the rewards of your mental and physical strength, you have to continue to invest in them. There is no going back to your old lifestyle, and that means you will have to commit to certain changes for the long haul.

- Fad diets are a total waste of time, as is excessive restriction of the things you love. What you are seeking is a new balance where you can indulge in moderation without compromising your progress towards mental or physical strength. Equally, it is important to admit that you will need to make changes if you want to see changes. Nutritional goals still have their place, and you cannot ignore the impact that food (and drink) can have on your strength.

- What works for you is what works. If you are achieving your strength goals and have found a balance and rhythm that suits you, don't feel the need to listen to any commentary on your diet. If you follow our guide to nutrition, you will be providing your body with everything it needs to progress, but the exact balance of how the calories and macronutrients are consumed is down to you.

- After you achieve some of your goals, you may find the people around you begin to react to the changed you in different ways. Remember that your progress can threaten others, and even people who love you can say and do things that might pull you down. Rise above and remember that you deserve to feel strong, no matter what. Anyone who wants to keep you from living strong is only showing their own weakness.

- Progress isn't linear and you've got to expect that you will have periods of plateauing and even breaks from your routine. Keep going, get back to your plan as soon as you can and never feel defeated – no one is perfect and it's a long-distance race not a sprint.

- Living in the present will help your mental health and relationships. While long-term goals are great to anchor your ambitions, make an effort to appreciate how far you have already come.

STEP SEVEN TO PHYSICAL STRENGTH: SLEEP IS FOR MORE THAN JUST BEAUTY

The power of rest, relaxation and a good night's sleep

Romane

When it comes to changing body composition, there's always been a disproportionate focus on the tearing of the muscle (the work you do in the gym) in comparison to the recovery of the muscle. To me, this seems really strange, especially when you consider that it's the recovery activity that actually increases the size of the myofibrils of the muscle. Rest and sleep are such important components of any fitness routine but are often overlooked because they're not quite as sexy as a gym selfie or posting about how much you've lifted. Several fundamental aspects of the muscle-building process happen exclusively during sleep, and without sufficient shut-eye you will struggle to fulfil your body's potential for muscle growth. Most tissue growth and repair happen at night, so if you're not getting proper sleep, you won't be maximising your muscle gains.

The most fundamental step in the muscle-building process during sleep is the release of human growth hormone (HGH). During our hours of slumber, HGH is released by the pituitary gland in pulses based on your body's internal clock or 'circadian rhythm'. The largest pulses occur before midnight, with some smaller pulses early in the morning, and these make up around 60–70 per cent of your overall HGH. Without HGH your body can't use the amino acids in the protein you eat to make muscle, and it also raises levels of insulin-like growth factor-1, another hormone involved in anabolic growth. It also has a direct relationship with the amount of fat that the body holds, as it stimulates lipolysis (the breakdown of fat) and seems to regulate fat deposition in tissue.

There is research that shows that non-REM sleep (the deepest periods of sleep) is most vital for muscle growth as it is during this time that your breathing is slower, deeper and your blood pressure drops. The brain is at rest with little activity, which means there is a bumper blood supply to your muscles, serving up those amino acids, oxygen and growth hormones. So it's not just the quantity of sleep that matters, but also the quality.

Lisa and I try to get eight hours of sleep every single night. We usually go to bed at 9pm, or at the latest 9.30pm. In the same way we know when we are dehydrated, if we don't get that proper sleep we will feel it very obviously in a physical sense the next day. It will impact our mood, our ability to complete our targets, and it will hit our overall results. Basically, it sucks. On balance, I would rather be hungry than tired, and I've already told you guys how hangry I get. When you're hungry it is frustrating, but you can still work out to an extent. But when you're tired you can't do anything. You can't train, you can't work, you can't think. And you definitely can't repair muscles effectively. Generally, sleep isn't a problem for us because we have such full-on days and we're so knackered when it gets to bedtime that we just fall asleep. So many studies have made the connection between an active lifestyle full of exercise and good-quality sleep, and exercise is often prescribed to help insomnia. For us, the relationship between the two is clear – better sleep means better workouts; better workouts mean better sleep. It's like the perfect feedback loop. And with the amount we do – all the training and the cardio and the work besides – we really need our sleep.

Because we get consistent sleep, we are in a good position to evaluate the effect it has on us physically. Recently, we stayed out late after a meal and didn't get to bed until around 2am, something that in our younger days wouldn't have been extraordinary. But the next day we both woke up feeling like we'd been on a massive bender, even though we hadn't drunk any alcohol. I like to go to bed early anyway as I'm an early riser, and Lisa and I love to walk early in the morning before the day starts. For us, it's a really special time and a great chance to reconnect while being active at the same time. Another benefit of sleep is that it helps to consolidate your memory, which can have a major impact on your form, leading to less chance of injury and increased effectiveness of every exercise you do in the gym. You are more accurate, your reaction time is much quicker and your overall performance improves markedly. For all the people looking for some magic supplement, try sleeping eight hours a night! It's literally one of the very best things you can do for gains.

Aside from these performance benefits, sleep is where you build your immune system. As you sleep, your body produces proteins called cytokines, which help fight infection and inflammation. Conversely, if your sleep is impaired, you will produce pro-inflammatory cytokines, which work against the immune system, putting you at a higher risk of getting sick. The classic story is that just before a holiday you're so stressed at work that you push yourself and compromise on sleep, then pick up a bug on the flight and spend most of your holiday feeling under the weather. Antibodies are also reduced when you have a lack of sleep, and sleep-deprived people who receive vaccinations will register far fewer antibodies than well-rested people who receive the same vaccine – something that is really relevant for our current situation. Sleep is just so vital to our overall well-being and health, so it is worth making a concerted effort to get it right.

This is why I always say that if you're feeling shattered, you should *not* try to power through. There's a lot of conflicting information out there on this, and somewhere there has been this message that if you want it enough, you will push yourself and your body no matter what. But that is just bullshit. If you need to sleep and rest, you need to sleep and rest; it is non-negotiable. Always listen to your body, that is the most important thing. If your body is telling you that it needs sleep, do not use caffeine to stay awake and do not force yourself to the mat that day. All you are doing is burning the candle at both ends, and in the long term, year on year, it's not going to be beneficial to your health at all.

The same principle goes for rest days. I get so many questions about how many rest days I take and whether or not I just carry on through. I always tell people that you have to listen to the signs your body is giving you, and more than that, try and refine how you tune into those messages. If I have a rest day, but still feel tired the next day, I'll take that day off too. I will never think, God, I've got to get to the gym, I've got to work through this fatigue. From experience I can tell you what will happen in that situation: you will hurt yourself. Over time, those rest days are not going to be detrimental to your overall progress. Remember, this is a lifestyle not a six-week plan. What *will* be detrimental is if you push yourself too hard when your body is telling you to rest. I've had some pretty serious injuries in the gym, and they've all been when I shouldn't have been training, so we definitely do not support any kind of gung-ho, train-till-you-break philosophy. Stop and think about it and you'll know that what we're saying is right. Slow, steady and consistent is the only way.

So how can you maximise your rest and sleep to make sure you are getting as much time for recovery and muscle tissue building as possible? Firstly, I'd recommend that you try to leave a good gap between training and bedtime. A side effect of high-intensity exercise is that the body gets a huge boost of energy through an increase in heart rate and the release of endorphins (which give you a high as they reduce the body's sensitivity to pain). But this surge of energy is likely to stop you from dropping off quickly, so it's best to leave a clear three-hour gap between high-intensity exercise and your bedtime.

Keeping a regular sleep schedule, where you go to sleep and wake up at roughly the same time every day, has been proven to offer the best quality of sleep. It's worth remembering that our bodies are biological clocks and if you can reinforce patterns across twenty-four hours, especially when it comes to sleep, your body will function at its best. It doesn't matter when you choose to wake up, as long as you wake up at the same time every day. Basically, the whole rhythm of wake and sleep is a series of processes with one step leading to the next. If you miss one, it's a like a house of cards – it all comes falling down. If you regularly go to sleep at 10pm, your brain is trained to release melatonin close to that time, and that makes you feel drowsy, ensuring you get a deeper sleep with multiple REM and non-REM cycles, both of which have benefits for muscle repair and growth. But if you decide to scroll your feed for ninety minutes when you get into bed, the brain has to postpone its release of melatonin and that causes a disruption to your circadian rhythm. When you finally put your phone down, you may find you're not tired at all, and when you do drop off, your quality of sleep may be poorer. It can even lead to insomnia.

During sleep, like any period of fasting, the body will engage in protein catabolism – breaking down muscle tissue into amino acids. That is why you will find many people recommending you drink a protein shake before bed. While that may be convenient for you, if you are able to eat a good amount of protein with your dinner, you will be just as well set up to maintain as much of your muscle mass as possible while continuing to gain overnight.

So never forget that there are two sides of the coin to gaining muscle: the work you do in the gym, and the rest and repair that happens afterwards. Both are equally important and require you to create a really solid lifestyle framework to maximise your potential.

LISA'S FITNESS PLAN

The following plan is divided into three phases. As with everything in this book, we absolutely recommend that you take it at your own pace. For those with some level of fitness training behind them, and who are perhaps already experienced with bodyweight movements, you may be able to phase up every month and find you are able to reach an advanced level by week twelve. For others, you might want to spend eight weeks or more on each phase, slowly increasing intensity and working on your form before you try and take the next step. It is entirely up to you and, as we have said before, it's not a race.

If you find you're fatiguing and can't manage to do all the reps of all the exercises, that is your body saying that it's not there yet and it's your job to respect that. Do not progress up a phase until you feel you can fairly comfortably manage the full exercises of the previous phase. For some people starting from scratch, with little experience of these kinds of movements, you might be working through phase one for three months until you feel like you can do a squat with a dumbbell, for example. We don't want to be prescriptive; everyone has their own fitness level and genetic individuality, which will have an impact on the speed at which they can move through these phases. Listen. To. Your. Body. I just cannot emphasise that enough. Whether it takes you twelve weeks or twelve months, this is the roadmap to take you from A to B. I also know nothing about your injury background or what your body has been through in the past, but you do. So be your own best supporter and take it as slow or as quick as your body can manage. It's three phases of progress – you need to get to a position of confidence with one phase before you move on to the next, and feeling that self-belief is key to everything that I teach.

PHASE ONE: BEGINNER

Below you will find a range of bodyweight exercises which are designed to get your body used to the kinds of movements you will need to progress into weightlifting. They are the true foundation of any lifting journey and the absolute cornerstone of success. The best thing about them is that they can all be done either at home or in a gym with limited equipment.

My advice for how to plan the different sessions are, as ever, to tailor it to your own body. This beginner plan has been designed to enable four days' training back to back, with a rest day or two until you feel ready to go again. It has been planned so that you will never exercise the same area of your body two days in a row, but you can also choose to rest for a day in between any of the workout days, if you prefer. As a beginner, you are going to be sore sometimes and you're going to hurt a lot more than someone who is more advanced in their training. That's just the way it is – we've all been there! If you still feel the DOMS (delayed onset muscle soreness), rest for another day then go back into it. So if you do the lower body on a Tuesday, say, then it gets to Thursday and your legs are still wrecking in a way that's painful for just regular everyday movements, rest for another day.

You might find either the upper body or the lower body sets easier – again, that is natural, but the key is to get to a place where you can comfortably do *all* of the exercises (unless you have specific injuries which prevent you making certain movements) before you progress on to the intermediate level.

Equipment needed: chair, table, something solid to step on to.

DAYS 1 & 3 LOWER BODY

Body Weight Squat
3 sets of 10 reps (reps meaning repetitions of the movement)
Ideal form:
1. Place your feet shoulder-width apart.
2. Ensure your toes point slightly outward in line with your knees.
3. Breathe in and brace your core (tense your stomach muscles to pull your ribs in and your lower tummy upwards).
4. Push your hips back and bend your knees as if you're sitting in an imaginary chair.
5. Push back up to standing through your heels.

Body Weight Glute Bridge
3 sets of 20 reps
Ideal form:
1. Lie down on your back and bring your knees up, with your feet on the floor, shoulder-width apart.
2. Keep your arms flat on the ground by your sides.
3. Keep your chin tucked in.

4. Push through your heels and lift your hips off the floor until your shoulders, hips and knees are aligned.

5. Squeeze your glute (bum) muscles at the top and slowly lower back down.

Static Lunge

3 sets of 10 reps per leg

Ideal form:

1. Start in a split stance position – one foot stretched ahead and the other stretched behind with your feet hip-width apart.

2. Place your hands on your hips.

3. Keep your spine in a neutral position (keep the three natural curves of your spine intact).

4. Lower the back knee down until it's 2.5-5cm (1–2 inches) off the ground.

5. Push off your front foot and repeat.

Body Weight Step Up

3 sets of 10 reps per leg

Ideal form:

1. Find something you can step up on to, which is around just under 20cm (7 inches) off the ground (once you get stronger in the movement, you can progress to using a chair).

2. Set the step in front of you.

3. Push through your heel and drive your body to stand on top of the step.

4. Focus on keeping your chest tall throughout the movement.

5. Step back to the floor safely.

Body Weight Donkey Kick

3 sets of 10 reps per leg

Ideal form:

1. Position yourself on your hands and knees with your knees under your hips and your hands under your shoulders.

2. Lift one leg so your thigh is parallel to the floor and your foot faces the ceiling, with the knee at a 90-degree angle.

3. Squeeze your glute (bum) muscles.

4. Lower back down.

DAYS 2 & 4 UPPER BODY

Press Up (on knees)

3 sets of 10 reps

Ideal form:

1. Kneel on the floor and place your hands shoulder-width (or just outside shoulder-width) apart.

2. Lower down and bring your elbows outward in line with the centre of your chest.

3. Stop when you are at a right angle, then push up with the palms and drive your elbows inward.

4. Don't lock out the elbows at the top; instead, keep them soft, ready for the next rep.

Body Weight Tricep Dip
3 sets of 10 reps
Ideal form:
1. Sit on the edge of a chair with your feet on the floor.
2. Place your hands behind you, directly under your shoulders with fingers facing your body.
3. Lower your body until the tops of your arms are facing the ceiling.
4. Push back up.

Body Weight Plank
2 sets of 15-second holds, (but start with what you can manage and build up from there)
Ideal form:
1. Start on your knees with your forearms on the floor, elbows under shoulders and feet hip-width apart.
2. Lift off your knees, keeping your body in a straight line.
3. Squeeze the glute (bum) muscles to maintain a strong posture.
4. Tense your stomach muscles tightly and hold for 15 seconds.

Reverse Crunch

3 sets of 10 reps

Ideal form:

1. Lie on your back with your arms by your sides.

2. Raise your legs with your knees bent at 90 degrees.

3. Breathe out and contract your abs, then bring your knees towards your chest and lift your hips and bum off the floor.

4. Lower back down.

Body Weight Inverted Row, with table

3 sets of 10 reps

Ideal form:

1. Lie on your back under a table.

2. Reach up to the edge of the table, holding your arms at 90 degrees to your shoulders.

3. Hold on to the edge of the table and pull yourself upwards. Don't worry if you can't pull yourself all the way up to start with – this will happen as you get stronger.

4. Lower back down.

PHASE TWO: INTERMEDIATE

Now we have laid the groundwork, it's time to hit the weight room. This is the moment when it gets real for a lot of people, and it can feel intimidating because if you haven't used machines before, there are all sorts of levers and cables and pulleys and many of the machines have multiple uses (especially the cable machines, for example). If you feel overwhelmed, I recommend watching some of my videos, where I perform all of the movements. Below, I've put together what I hope are some really clear, succinct instructions on each exercise. I haven't given a full run-down on how to adjust each machine, simply because they all are slightly different. If in doubt, ask a PT, though my rule of thumb is to always load the very lowest weight until you are 100 per cent certain of form, so you have a bit of licence to experiment if you're not feeling totally confident with your positioning on a machine or how the movement works. It isn't rocket science, but that doesn't mean there isn't a lot to learn at first.

This programme is a five-day workout training split of each muscle group, meaning that you could go five days straight if you aren't horribly sore, then take a rest day. You know what I'm going to say next – take it at your own pace and listen to your body. I'm totally aware that you may not have five opportunities to work out in a single week. Just follow the pattern outlined with the time you have and you will make progress, albeit more slowly the more the sessions are spread out.

This is a big step up for most people, even if you have a pretty good fitness level from other disciplines, so take time to hone your movements and enjoy the process. This is where you will probably fall in love with weightlifting and are going to start seeing some real results in your strength, so it can be an exciting time. But keep reminding yourself that it's still only the start of your journey, so even if you get really pumped up, keep safe and sensible with what you're lifting; the last thing you want to do is get an injury at this stage. I would recommend a minimum of four to six weeks before attempting to go on to the next phase.

DAY 1 BACK

Barbell Bent Over Row
3 sets of 12 reps
Equipment needed: barbell, weights
A barbell is a long bar with weights at each end. Start with a fixed barbell as they generally start at a low weight, for example 7.5g, and that will enable you to practise with your form before progressing up in weight.
Ideal form:
1. Stand behind the barbell with a flat back.
2. Hinge at the hips and grip the bar at just outside shoulder-width, keeping your arms extended.
3. Brace your core muscles and squeeze your shoulder blades together as you row the bar in towards your sternum. Drive

your feet into the floor as you pick up the bar. Keep your hips high and your torso almost parallel to the floor.

4. Extend your arms back down to the starting position with control.

Cable Row

3 sets of 12 reps

Equipment needed: cable machine

A weighted horizontal cable machine with bench or footplates can be a stand-alone piece of equipment or part of a multi-gym machine. There are various attachments you can use with cable – here we are using a V-bar grip, which are two small handles placed in a V-shape to create a tight grip and target the latissimus dorsi (lats) muscles. Start at the lowest weight available, testing your strength and increasing over time.

Ideal form:

1. Attach a V-bar grip to the machine.

2. Initiate the movement by pulling the cable in towards the bottom of your rib cage.

3. Keep the elbows tucked in.

4. At the top of the rep, squeeze the shoulder blades together for one second.

5. Try not to only pull with your biceps; really feel the movement and think about the muscle you're working.

Lat Pull Down

3 sets of 12 reps

Equipment: lat pull down machine

You may recognise this one from the wide bar hanging over a bench, though there are various attachments which can be used here too. Start at the lowest weight available, testing your strength and increasing over time.

Ideal form:

1. Keep your torso upright.

2. Initiate the movement by squeezing your lats to pull your shoulders down (a movement known as scapular depression) and lower the bar slightly.

3. Retract the shoulder blades as you reach the bottom of the rep.

4. Release the weight back up to the starting position with control.

Single Arm Dumbbell Row

3 sets of 12 reps per arm

Equipment: bench and dumbbell

Ideal form:

1. Place one knee and one hand on a bench. Anchor your other foot on the floor and keep your back flat in a tabletop position.

2. Holding the dumbbell with the opposite arm, initiate the movement by driving your elbow up towards the hip, keeping your elbow tucked in.

Assisted Pull Up
3 sets of 10 reps
Equipment: assisted pull up machine
This machine has an overhead bar with a platform beneath for you to kneel on. Start with a heavy weight (the heavier the weight, the more resistance it will give you, helping you to achieve the movement).
Ideal form:
1. Stand on the platform.
2. Grab hold of the bar outside shoulder-width apart.
3. Initiate the movement by pulling the shoulder blades down (scapular depression).
4. Retract the shoulder blades as you pull up and drive the elbows into 'pockets'.
5. Control yourself by keeping your chest high and core braced.
6. Lower back down.

DAY 2 QUADS/ GLUTES /CALVES

Barbell Squat
4 sets of 10–12 reps

Equipment: barbell, weights, squat rack

Start with a fixed barbell before progressing on to a squat rack, as these generally start at a low weight.

Ideal form:

1. If the weight is light enough, shoulder press the bar up and over the traps, on to the top of your shoulders.
2. Set up for your squat by placing your feet shoulder-width apart.
3. Point your toes slightly outward in line with your knees.
4. Retract your shoulder blades to keep your shoulders back.
5. Take a breath in and brace your core.
6. Push your hips backward and bend your knees as if you are sitting in an imaginary chair.
7. Push back up through your heels.

Leg Press

3 sets of 10–12 reps

Equipment: leg press machine

A seated machine with a foot plate set at 90 degrees for your feet to push against. Start at the lowest weight available, testing your strength and increasing over time.

Ideal form:

1. Sit the hips back into the seat, then place the feet just inside shoulder-width apart on the footplate.

2. Push the weight slowly up and unrack safely, bracing the core while grabbing on to the handles for support.

3. Lower the weight with control, without rounding your lower back.

4. Push up through your heels but don't fully lock (straighten) your legs at the top.

5. Ensure your knees aren't caving inward during the exercise.

Leg Extension
4 sets of 12 reps

Equipment: leg extension machine

Another seated machine with a column-shaped leg pad on a hinged bar in front of the seat. Start at the lowest weight available, testing your strength and increasing over time.

Ideal form:

1. Adjust the machine to place the pad just above your ankles and lock your hands on the grips where it feels natural.

2. Align the backs of your knees with the edge of the seat.

3. Keep your glutes and hips fixed into the back of the seat at all times.

4. Raise your legs, extending them as high as possible towards the ceiling and keeping the toes pointed forward.

5. Lower the legs back down.

Hip Thrust

3 sets of 12 reps

Equipment: bench, dumbbell, exercise mat

Ideal form:

1. Align the bottom of your shoulder blades with the edge of a bench (ideal height is 30–45cm/12–18 inches, relative to each person).

2. Place your feet shoulder-width apart. Play around with your foot positioning to see what suits you best. Toes can be slightly flared out or face forward.

3. Adjust your feet so your shins are vertical for optimal glute activation. Feet further forward = recruit more hamstrings; feet further backward = recruit more quads.

4. As you extend your hips, push your knees out and push through your heels, making sure your body is parallel to the floor.

5. Keep your chin tucked in or your head neutral.

6. Reach full hip extension by squeezing the glutes and making sure your shoulders, hips and knees are in line.

7. Now you have your positioning set up, incorporate a dumbbell by placing it on the pubic bone with an exercise mat underneath for comfort and repeat the above steps.

Romanian Deadlift (RDL)

3 sets of 12 reps

Equipment: barbell, weights, squat rack

Start with a fixed barbell before progressing on to a squat rack, as these generally start at a low weight.

Ideal form:

1. Place the bar on to a bench.

2. Grasp the bar just outside your legs.

3. Pick the bar up and step back a couple of steps.

4. Retract your shoulder blades slightly.

5. Push your hips back and hinge forward from your hips, keeping your back flat.

6. Keep the bar close to your body and let it slide down your legs to just below the knee.

7. Push your hips forward and come back to the starting position.

Seated Calf Raise

3 sets of 20 reps

Equipment: seated calf raise machine

A seated machine with a foot platform below two knee pads. Start at the lowest weight available, testing your strength and increasing over time.

Ideal form:

1. Place your knees under the pads and place your toes on the platform.

2. Unrack the weight slowly (often by releasing a lever, but check the specific machine), keeping your toes pointed

forward and slowly bringing the weight down on to the knees.

3. Push up through the toes and contract hard at the top.

4. Bring toes back down to the starting position.

DAY 3 SHOULDERS

Seated Dumbbell Shoulder Press
3 sets of 12 reps
Equipment: bench, dumbbells
Start at the lowest weight available, testing your strength and increasing over time.

Ideal form:
1. Hold a dumbbell in each hand at the shoulders with your palms facing away.
2. Drive the weight above your head but don't fully extend the elbows at the top.
3. Bring the arms back down to the starting position.

Dumbbell Lat Raise
3 sets of 12 reps
Equipment: dumbbells
Start at the lowest weight available, testing your strength and increasing over time.

Ideal form:
1. Stand upright with your shoulders back.
2. Hold the dumbbells at your sides, elbows slightly bent, and lift your arms outward like wings, leading with your elbows, aiming for the dumbbells to stop level with your shoulders.
3. Keep your wrists below your elbows at all times.

Dumbbell Front Raise
3 sets of 12 reps
Equipment: bench, dumbbells
Start at the lowest weight available, testing your strength and increasing over time.
Ideal form:
1. Sit on a bench.
2. Hold the dumbbells at the sides of your body.
3. Raise both arms out in front of you, to shoulder height, keeping your palms facing down.
4. Avoid leaning back or swinging as you raise.

Dumbbell Arnold Press
3 sets of 12 reps
Equipment: bench, dumbbells
Start at the lowest weight available, testing your strength and increasing over time.

Ideal form:

1. Sit on a bench.

2. Hold the dumbbells in front of the shoulders, with your palms facing in.

3. Initiate the movement by bringing the elbows out to the sides and rotating your palms as you press the dumbbells over your head until they are facing outward.

Reverse Pec Dec

3 sets of 12 reps

Equipment: pec machine, adjusted into the reverse position

Start at the lowest weight available, testing your strength and increasing over time.

Ideal form:

1. Sit facing into the machine and position the handles in front of you.

2. Place your hands on the inside handles.

3. Push the handles outward and back together as you contract your back and squeeze your shoulder blades tightly.

DAY 4 CHEST & ARMS

Barbell Bench Press

3 sets of 10 reps

Equipment: barbell, weights, squat rack

Start with a fixed barbell before progressing on to a squat rack, as these generally start at a low weight.

Ideal form:

1. Lie back on a bench, keeping the natural curve in your spine to help with power and to protect your shoulders.
2. Grip the barbell overhead with your hands just outside shoulder-width apart.
3. Take a deep breath in and slowly lower the bar down to touch your chest, while pressing your feet into the floor.
4. Push up as you breathe out.

Incline Bench Press

3 sets of 10 reps

Equipment: barbell, weights, squat rack

Start with a fixed barbell before progressing on to a squat rack, as these generally start at a low weight.

Ideal form:

1. Lie back on an incline bench (a regular bench set at an incline angle).
2. Grip the barbell overhead, just outside shoulder-width apart.
3. Retract your shoulder blades, take a deep breath in and let the bar descend.
4. Let the bar touch the sternum and push back up.

Standing Cable Fly

3 sets of 12 reps

Equipment: cable fly machine

You'll see two handles attached to a cable pulley on either side of a machine. Start at the lowest weight available, testing your strength and increasing over time.

Ideal form:

1. Set the attachments at around shoulder height.

2. Hold the handles with a neutral grip and stand in a split stance with your front leg bent at the knee and your back leg straight.

3. Keep a slight bend in the elbows and pull forward to meet at the sternum.

4. Allow the arms to open fully and return to the starting position.

Barbell Bicep Curl

3 sets of 12 reps

Equipment: barbell, weights

Use a fixed barbell as these generally start at a low weight.

Ideal form:

1. Grasp the bar with your hands shoulder-width apart, palms facing up to the ceiling.

2. Keep your elbows pinched into your sides.

3. Contract the biceps as you curl the bar up to your chest.

4. Lower it back down with control.

Cable Bicep Curl

3 sets of 12 reps

Equipment: cable machine, cable bar

Start at the lowest weight available, testing your strength and increasing over time.

Ideal form:

1. Attach a bar to the cable.

2. Keep your elbows pinched into your sides.

3. Contract the biceps as you curl the bar up.

4. Lower it back down with control.

DAY 5: HAMSTRINGS/ GLUTES/ CALVES

Sumo Kettlebell Deadlift

3 sets of 10–12 reps

Equipment: kettlebell

Start at the lowest weight available, testing your strength and increasing over time.

Ideal form:

1. Take a wide stance with feet turned out.

2. Push the hips back and lean forward slightly so your shoulders are aligned over the kettlebell.

3. Grasp the kettlebell with palms facing inward.

4. Drive through your feet and push off.

5. Once you reach full hip extension, reverse the movement by pushing the hips backward.

Hip Thrust

4 sets of 12 reps

See Day 2, page 273

Lying Leg Curl

3 sets of 12 reps

Equipment: lying leg curl machine

Start at the lowest weight available, testing your strength and increasing over time.

Ideal form:

1. Lie down on your front and position the pad just above the backs of your ankles and hold on to the handles.

2. Use your hamstrings to pull the weight upwards towards your bum, making sure your hips stay touching the bench.

3. Slowly release the weight back down.

Stiff Leg Kettlebell Deadlift

3 sets of 12 reps

Equipment: kettlebell

Start at the lowest weight available, testing your strength and increasing over time.

Ideal form:

1. Stand up with the kettlebell positioned in front of your feet.
2. Push your hips back and hinge forward to grasp the kettlebell (palms facing inward), keeping a slight bend in the knees and your back straight until your torso is nearly parallel with the floor.
3. Lift the kettlebell off the floor, keeping your core tight.
4. Keep your back straight and the kettlebell close to your legs until you reach full hip extension (standing up straight).
5. Squeeze the glutes and reverse the movement by pushing the hips back in to lower the kettlebell.

Seated Calf Raise
3 sets of 20 reps
See Day 2, page 274

PHASE THREE: ADVANCED

Well done for sticking with it and getting this far! Hopefully you are starting to feel the benefits of your hard work, and if you're anything like me you will be getting hooked on the weightlifting high. This final phase incorporates a range of more advanced movements, but also gives you different techniques to help increase the target muscle's time under tension, which is key for growth. There are several exercises here which you will have done before if you've progressed through the previous two phases, but it's the approach and intensity that differ.

A few techniques

Partials – A partial rep is a limited-range-of-motion movement that mimics a full-range-of-motion movement, keeping the constant tension leading to high levels of metabolic stress, helping to promote muscle growth. You will always aim to lift a lighter weight on partials because it's so intense. For example, on a hip thrust, instead of doing a full rep from bottom to top, you would go from the top, halfway down, and back up to the top.

3 Fast Reps, 3 Slow Reps – Complete three reps at a faster pace with control, and the next three really slowly. Again, you will aim to lift a lighter weight as it is very intense. Slower reps cause your muscles to experience more TUT (time under tension), helping to promote muscle growth.

Iso Hold – An isometric hold is where you reach a position and hold it for the desired amount of time, causing tension in the muscles.

283

Negative – Control the tempo of the repetition and slow down the eccentric (lowering) phase of the lift for the specified time, keeping the tension constant to help promote muscle growth.

Superset – Perform two exercises back to back without rest.

Below is another five-day workout training spilt of each muscle group, which you can follow on five consecutive days or incorporate rest days in between depending on your available gym time and rest requirements. As you phase up, you're probably going to feel the intensity of the DOMs again, so take it slowly and enjoy watching your body transform to strong!

DAY 1 BACK

A) Superset: Straight Arm Pull Down with Lat Pull Down
3 sets of 10 reps
Equipment: cable machine, wide bar
Start at the lowest weight available, testing your strength and increasing over time.
Ideal form:
1. Position the attachment at the top of the cable.
2. Attach a wide bar to the cable.

3. Hold the bar with your palms facing down, shoulder-width apart.

4. Lean forward slightly.

5. Initiate the movement by pulling your shoulder blades down and pulling the bar into your thighs.

6. Keep the spine neutral throughout.

7. Continue on to part B of the superset.

B) Superset Lat Pull Down
3 sets of 10 reps, to be completed after part A
See Phase 2, Day 1, page 269

Cable Row
3 sets of 12 reps
See Phase 2, Day 1, page 268

Single Arm Dumbbell Row
3 sets of 12 reps
See Phase 2, Day 1, page 269

Body Weight Chin Up
3 sets of 8 reps with 3-second negative
Equipment: pull up bar
Ideal form:
1. Initiate the movement by pulling the shoulder blades down (scapular depression).

2. Retract the shoulder blades as you pull up and drive the elbows into 'pockets'.

3. Keep your knees bent.

4. Initiate the movement by retracting your shoulder blades and pulling your body up until your chin becomes aligned with the bar.

5. Pause for two seconds and slowly lower back down.

DAY 2 QUADS/ GLUTES/ CALVES

Barbell Squat

4 sets of 10–12 reps

Equipment: barbell, weights, squat rack

Begin by lifting the bar alone, then add weight to each end of the bar. Start at the lowest weight available, testing your strength and increasing over time.

Ideal form:

1. Set the bar on a squat rack at just below shoulder height, as it is going to go over your head and sit across your shoulders.

2. Come below the bar in a split stance, one foot in front of the other. Rest the bar across the shoulders and step back away from the rack.

3. Set up for your squat by placing your feet shoulder-width apart with your toes pointing outward in line with your knees.

4. Retract your shoulder blades to keep your shoulders back.

5. Take a breath in and brace your core.

6. Push your hips backward as if you are sitting in an imaginary chair.

7. Push back up through your heels.

Leg Press

1 set of 12 reps

Followed by 2 sets of 10 reps with 3-second negative

See Phase 2, Day 2, page 271

A) Superset: Leg Extension with Elevated Heel Goblet Squat

3 sets of 10 reps

See Phase 2, Day 2, page 272

Continue on to part B of the superset.

B) Superset: Elevated Heel Goblet Squat

3 sets of 10 reps

Equipment: dumbbell or kettlebell, 5kg incline plate or wedge to elevate your heels

Start at the lowest weight available, testing your strength and increasing over time.

Ideal form:

1. Grab the kettlebell or dumbbell.

2. Elevate your heels on a 5kg incline plate or wedge.

3. Position your feet about shoulder-width apart.

4. Hold the weight close to your chest and keep your elbows pinched in.

5. Lower down and push back up through your heels then straight back down again.

Hip Thrust

2 sets of 12 partial reps

Followed by 1 set of 12 reps with 2-second iso hold

Followed by 1 set of 20 reps

Equipment: hip thrust machine

A seated machine with a column-shaped pad across the front of the hips. Start at the lowest weight available, testing your strength and increasing over time.

Ideal form:

1. Raise the bar high enough to roll it across your legs. Rest the bottom of the shoulder blades on a padded bench.

2. Position the feet so your knees will end up in a right angle when at the top of the movement and the shins are vertical.

3. Push up through your heels, thrusting your hips upwards until you reach full hip extension.

4. Keep looking forward with the chin tucked in.

5. Make sure your knees don't cave inward. Squeeze the glutes at the top.

6. Slowly lower your hips back to the original position.

DAY 3 SHOULDERS

Barbell Military Press

3 sets of 8–10 reps

Equipment: barbell, weights

Start at the lowest weight available, testing your strength and increasing over time.

Ideal form:

1. Position the barbell below shoulder height on a rack.

2. Place your feet shoulder-width apart and place your hands at (or just outside of) shoulder-width with a pronated grip (palms facing towards hips) on the bar.

3. Unrack the barbell while keeping the spine in a neutral position.

4. Push the barbell upwards into press movement.

5. Keeping the wrists tight, lower the barbell down with elbows out and in line with the middle of the chest.

6. Lower until the elbows hit a right angle.

7. Keep the core braced and engaged and the spine tight throughout the movement.

Cable Lying Crucifix Lat Raise

2 sets of 12 reps

1 set of 15 partial reps

Equipment: cable machine, incline bench

Start at the lowest weight available, testing your strength and increasing over time.

Ideal form:

1. Pull the bench close to the cable stack.

2. Sit on a flat bench facing the stack.

2. Set the cables just above the legs.

3. Grab on to the handles with the hands crossed over, lay back on the bench and pull up and out as hard as you can.

4. Release the weight slowly.

A) *Superset: Cable Front Raise with Rope, with Steering Wheels*

3 sets of 10 reps

Equipment: cable machine, rope

Start at the lowest weight available, testing your strength and increasing over time.

Ideal form:

1. Adjust the cable machine to the bottom setting, as close to the floor as possible, and attach a rope to the pulley.

2. Stand upright, facing away from the machine with your shoulders back.

3. Hold the rope in front of you with palms facing inward and elbows pinched into the sides.

4. Lift the arms out and up towards the ceiling until you reach shoulder height.

5. Control the weight as you lower it down.

6. Continue on to part B of the superset.

B) *Superset Steering Wheels*

3 sets of 10 reps

Equipment: gym plate

Start at the lowest weight available, testing your strength and increasing over time.

Ideal form:

1. Place your feet shoulder-width apart.

2. Keep your core braced and engaged as this will help to stabilise you.

3. Raise the plate out in front of you.

4. Steer from the 3 o'clock to the 9 o'clock position.

Dumbbell Arnold Press

3 sets of 12 reps

See Phase 2, Day 3, page 276

Cable Face Pull

3 sets of 12 reps

Equipment: cable machine, rope attachment

Ideal form:

1. Attach a rope to the cable pulley.

2. Start with your arms straight out in front of you with your palms facing downwards.

3. Pull the rope towards your face, keeping your elbows up high and contracting the rear deltoid muscles.

DAY 4 CHEST & ARMS

Bench Press
3 sets of 10 reps
Equipment: bench, barbell, barbell rack, weights
Start at the lowest weight available, testing your strength and increasing over time.
Ideal form:
1. Lie back on to a bench, keeping the natural curve in your spine to help with power and to protect your shoulders.
2. Grip the barbell overhead with your hands just wider than shoulder-width apart.
3. Take a deep breath in and slowly lower the bar down to touch your chest, while pressing your feet into the floor.
4. Push up as you breathe out.

Incline Bench Press
3 sets of 10 reps
Equipment: incline bench, barbell, barbell rack, weights
Start at the lowest weight available, testing your strength and increasing over time.

Ideal form:

1. Lie back on an incline bench (a regular bench set at an incline angle).

2. Set your hands on the barbell overhead, just outside shoulder-width apart.

3. Retract your shoulder blades, take a deep breath and lower the bar.

4. Let the bar touch the sternum and push back up.

Standing Cable Fly
3 sets of 12 reps
See Phase 2, Day 4, page 279

Barbell Bicep Curl 21s
2 sets of 21 reps
7 reps bottom to halfway up
7 reps top to halfway down
7 full reps
See Phase 2, Day 4, page 279

Cable Bicep Curl
3 sets of 12 reps
3 fast reps followed by 3 slow reps, repeat twice
See Phase 2, Day 4, page 280

DAY 5: HAMSTRINGS/ GLUTES/ CALVES

Barbell Glute Bridge
3 sets of 12 reps with 2-second iso hold
Equipment: barbell, weights, barbell pad
Start at the lowest weight available, testing your strength and increasing over time.

Ideal form:
1. Start in a supine position on the floor.
2. Attach a barbell pad.
3. Roll the bar over your thighs and align it above your pubic bone.
4. Bridge your hips by squeezing your glutes for 2 seconds and driving your heels into the floor.
5. Lower your hips back to the starting position.

Hip Thrust Pyramid
1 set of 12 reps
1 set of 10 reps
1 set of 8 reps
(This is the pyramid part!)
Followed by 1 set of 20 partial reps
See Phase 3, Day 2, page 288

Seated Leg Curl
2 sets of 12 reps with 2-second hold and 3-second negative

1 set of 15 reps

Equipment: leg curl machine

Start at the lowest weight available, testing your strength and increasing over time.

Ideal Form:

1. Sit on the machine and make sure the seat back is upright. You are going to be bringing the padded bar downwards rather than upwards, as with the leg extension exercise we worked on in Phase 2, Day 2, page 272.

2. Lock the knee guard down and hold on to the handles.

3. Hinge your legs downwards at the knees.

Stiff Leg Barbell Deadlift

3 sets of 12 reps

Equipment: barbell, weights

Increase the weight only when you feel comfortable.

Ideal Form:

1. Standing up, position the barbell in front of your feet.

2. Push your hips back, hinge forward and grasp the barbell with an overhand grip, keeping a slight bend in the knees and the back straight until your torso is nearly parallel with the floor (this is your starting position).

3. Lift the barbell off the floor, keeping your core tight and the barbell close to your legs until you get to full hip extension (standing up straight).

Squeeze the glutes and reverse the movement by pushing the hips back in to lower the barbell.

Seated Calf Raise
2 sets of 20 reps
1 set of 15 partial reps
See Phase 2, Day 2, page 274

Phases Overview

PHASE ONE

DAY 1 & 3 Lower Body	
Body Weight Squat	3 x 10
Body Weight Glute Bridge	3 x 20
Static Lunge	3 x 10
Body Weight Step Up	3 x 10 each leg
Body Weight Donkey Kick	3 x 10 each leg

DAY 2 & 4 Upper Body	
Press Up (on knees)	3 x 10
Body Weight Tricep Dip	3 x 10
Body Weight Plank	2 x 15 seconds
Reverse Crunch	3 x 10
Body Weight Inverted Row, with table	3 x 10

PHASE TWO

Back	
Barbell Bent Over Row	3 x 12
Cable Row	3 x 12
Lat Pull Down	3 x 12
Single Arm Dumbbell Row	3 x 12 each arm
Assisted Pull Up	3 x 10

Quads/Glutes/Calves	
Barbell Squat	4 x 10–12
Leg Press	3 x 10–12
Leg Extension	4 x 12
Hip Thrust	3 x 12
Romanian Deadlift (RDL)	3 x 12
Seated Calf Raise	3 x 20

Shoulders	
Seated Dumbbell Shoulder Press	3 x 12
Dumbbell Lat Raise	3 x 12
Dumbbell Front Raise	3 x 12
Dumbbell Arnold Press	3 x 12
Reverse Pec Dec	3 x 12

Chest & Arms	
Barbell Bench Press	3 x 10
Incline Bench Press	3 x 10

Standing Cable Fly	3 x 12
Barbell Bicep Curl	3 x 12
Cable Bicep Curl	3 x 12

Hams/Glutes/Calves	
Sumo Kettlebell Deadlift	3 x 10–12
Hip Thrust	4 x 12
Lying Leg Curl	3 x 12
Stiff Leg Kettlebell Deadlift	3 x 12
Seated Calf Raise	3 x 20

PHASE THREE

Back	
Superset: Straight Arm Pull Down with Lat Pull Down	3 x 10; 3 x 10
Cable Row	3 x 12
Single Arm Dumbbell Row	3 x 12
Body Weight Chin Up	3 x 8 with 3-second negative

Quads/Glutes/Calves	
Barbell Squat	4 x 10–12
Leg Press	1 x 12 2 x 10 with 3-second negative

Superset: Leg Extension with Elevated Heel Goblet Squat	3 x 10; 3 x 10
Hip Thrust	2 x 12 partial 1 x 12 with 2-second iso hold 1 x 20
Romanian Deadlift	3 x 12

Shoulders	
Barbell Military Press	3 x 8–10
Cable Lying Crucifix Lat Raise	2 x 12 1 x 15 partial
Superset: Cable Front Raise with Rope, with Steering Wheels	3 x 10; 3 x 10
Dumbbell Arnold Press	3 x 12
Cable Face Pull	3 x 12

Chest & Arms	
Bench Press	3 x 10
Incline Bench Press	3 x 10
Standing Cable Fly	3 x 12
Barbell Bicep Curl 21s	2 x 21 (7 reps bottom to halfway up; 7 reps top to halfway down; 7 full)

Cable Bicep Curl	3 x 12 (3 fast reps + 3 slow reps)

Hams/Glutes/Calves	
Barbell Glute Bridge	3 x 12 with 2-second iso hold
Hip Thrust Pyramid	1 x 12 1 x 10 1 x 8 1 x 20 partial
Seated Leg Curl	2 x 12 with 2-second hold and 3-second negative 1 x 15
Stiff Leg Barbell Deadlift	3 x 12
Seated Calf Raise	2 x 20 1 x 15 partial

ACKNOWLEDGEMENTS

I would like to thank my family and friends for always encouraging me during my journey and always being so supportive in everything I do. To my amazing followers who support and put their trust in me – without you I wouldn't be where I am today. To Katherine Ormerod, who helped Romane and me tell our story, thank you for everything. And finally, a big thank you to everyone at Century, Penguin Random House for their support with this book, in particular: Ben Brusey, Hope Butler, Amy Musgrave, Callum Crute, Laurie Ip Fung Chun, Linda Hodgson and Sarah Bennie.

INDEX

LL indicates Lisa Lanceford.

husband, first meets 67–72
    see also Lanceford,
    Romane
Instagram and *see* Instagram
jobs/working life 3, 14, 52–6,
    61, 128–9, 172, 202
living in the present, focus
    on 241–2, 246
meeting new people, anxiety
    over 134–5
romantic relationships 3,
    56–63
school/education and 3, 11,
    12–14, 15–16, 17, 31,
    53, 94, 130–1, 172–3,
    177–8, 195, 202, 203–4,
    207
self-belief, development of
    129–33
setbacks and pauses 232–40
social circle, on importance
    of 52–73
social media career, anxieties
    associated with 134–45
social media career, begins
    64–7

social media product sales,
    on 139–43, 168–72
STRNG app and *see*
    STRNG app
support network 230–2
thigh gap 17, 32
voice, volume of 55–6, 133
weight 21, 99–101, 124
weight room, first enters
    23–5
when to take yourself
    seriously, on 127–50
Lanceford, Romane
    calories, on 118–26
    childhood 70
    compromises to achieve
        things in the gym, on
        making 227–8
    Dubai, move to 206
    emotional overeating,
        history of 224
    gratitude 242, 243
    haters and 231, 232
    hydration, on 182–9
    injuries, on 210–19
    LL first meets 67–72

short cuts 92–3, 114

sit-ups 176

six packs 22, 23

skeletal muscle 38

sleep 247–55

  circadian rhythm 249

  human growth hormone
    (HGH) and 249

  immune system and 251–2

  muscle recovery and 248–9

  non-REM sleep 249–50

  performance benefits of 251

  'powering through' and 252

  protein catabolism and 255

  rest days and 252–3

  schedule 254

  training and bedtime, time
    between 253–4

social circle

  choosing 52–73

  Instagram and 64–8

  romantic relationships
    57–65, 67–72

  seeking out relationships with
    people whose values
    align with your own 72–3

workplace and 53–7, 128–9

social media 2, 15, 18, 22–3,
  65, 94

  age and success on 203–5

  attitudes towards careers
    built through 134–8

  expectation and 193–6, 203–4

  fakery on 114, 137–44, 164,
    168–71, 174, 178

  humour, using on 145–8

  'likes' 148–9

  negative body comments on
    26–8, 31–2

  negative messages on 139–43

  nutritional advice on 225

  partnerships, commercial
    169, 171, 178

  product sales on 139–42,
    169–71, 178

  suggestive, sexual comments
    on 30–1

  vanity levels on 147

  workout videos on 31, 110,
    126, 132, 176, 266

  see also Facebook and
    Instagram